PRECISION

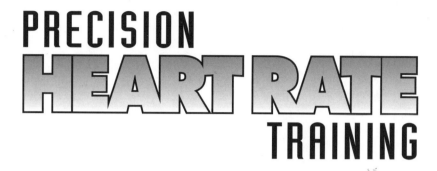

HEART RATE
TRAINING

Edmund R. Burke, PhD
University of Colorado at Colorado Springs

Editor

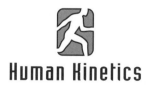

Human Kinetics

Library of Congress Cataloging-in-Publication Data

Precision heart rate training / Edmund R. Burke, editor.
    p.   cm.
   ISBN 0-88011-770-2
   1. Aerobic exercises.   2. Heart rate monitoring.   3. Athletes-
-Health and hygiene.   4. Exercise–Physiological aspects.
I. Burke, Ed, 1949-
RC1236.H43P74   1998
613.7'1–dc21

                                                     97-44079
                                                       CIP

ISBN: 0-88011-770-2

Photos on pages 49 and 61 © Ken Lee. Photo on page 112 courtesy of John Lash. Photo on page 124 courtesy of Frank Fedel. Photos on pages 149 and 155 by Tom Roberts. Photo on page 194 courtesy of Jim Dotter. All other photos courtesy of Polar Electro, Inc.

Developmental Editor: Marni Basic; **Assistant Editors:** Henry V. Woolsey and Katy M. Patterson; **Copyeditor:** Joyce Sexton; **Proofreader:** Myla Smith; **Graphic Designer:** Nancy Rasmus; **Graphic Artist:** Angela K. Snyder; **Photo Editor:** Boyd LaFoon; **Cover Designer:** Jack Davis; **Photographer (cover):** © POLAR/John Mireles; **Illustrator:** Craig Ronto; **Printer:** Versa.

Human Kinetics books are available at special discounts for bulk purchase. Special editions or book excerpts can also be created to specification. For details, contact the Special Sales Manager at Human Kinetics.

Printed in the United States of America   10 9 8 7 6 5 4 3 2 1

Human Kinetics
Web site: http://www.humankinetics.com/

United States: Human Kinetics
P.O. Box 5076
Champaign, IL 61825-5076
1-800-747-4457
e-mail: humank@hkusa.com

Canada: Human Kinetics, Box 24040
Windsor, ON N8Y 4Y9
1-800-465-7301 (in Canada only)
e-mail: humank@hkcanada.com

Europe: Human Kinetics, P.O. Box IW14
Leeds LS16 6TR, United Kingdom
(44) 1132 781708
e-mail: humank@hkeurope.com

Australia: Human Kinetics
57A Price Avenue
Lower Mitcham, South Australia 5062
(088) 277 1555
e-mail: humank@hkaustralia.com

New Zealand: Human Kinetics
P.O. Box 105-231, Auckland 1
(09) 523 3462
e-mail: humank@hknewz.com

CONTENTS

FOREWORD

In the early 1980s, I was presenting a clinic in Florida on training and racing to a group of endurance athletes. At the conclusion, one of the triathletes asked, "How important is it to monitor heart rate during my higher-intensity training days?" I replied, "Well, it's nearly impossible to accurately record heart rate during intense activity." He persisted, saying, "I've noticed that during late-afternoon runs, my heart rate seems to be extraordinarily high, my breathing is labored, I'm sweating profusely, and I just can't hold my pace." I realized that my next explanation was limited, but with some confidence, I responded, "Your heart rate is naturally higher because of the humidity and the 90° outside temperature, and concurrently your respirations go up and ultimately your pace slows down." Not exactly a textbook response; frankly, I didn't know the answer. However, a few years later, with the introduction of heart rate monitors, I certainly would have been more prepared to answer his questions.

Even though I had exposure to heart rate monitors over a decade ago, I didn't train with one until 1991. I had stopped racing for a couple of years because of injuries and started looking at the possibility of racing at a top level again as I neared the age of forty.

As a new training "tool," the heart rate monitor allowed me the luxury of controlling the intensity and duration of my workouts. I was wrestling not only with middle age but also with having a family, moving to high altitude in Colorado, and trying to allocate my training time. It was vital to monitor my heart rate during all of my workouts.

Fortunately, my best times (even though I was not victorious) in the Ironman came at 40 and 42 years of age. I attributed my performances to good genes and to the routine scrutiny of my heart rate. When I was overstressed physically or psychologically, the monitor became my barometer. As I discovered during 20 years of training, it was shortsighted to look solely at my perceived exertion and pace as true measurements for assessing the intensity of my workouts. Heart rate training allowed me the opportunity to look at the following variables and questions:

- Is an elevated heart rate in the morning due to overtraining, work, family commitments, lack of sleep, or simply advancing age?
- Exercising at altitudes of 6,000 to 10,000 feet is a tad tiring! What heart rate intensity can I maintain?
- How much time is needed between workouts to adequately recover?
- Can speed and power be developed at higher altitudes? Is the intensity the same as at sea level, and should my recovery time be shorter or longer?
- How can I maximize my time, allowing for a heart-rate-based progression in training as well as adequate recovery times?

My questions about training were answered by regularly using the heart rate monitor. In *Precision Heart Rate Training*, you will have the opportunity to determine and evaluate your heart rate load for yourself and to learn some surprising facts. For example: The person with a high heart rate is not necessarily the fittest athlete. Two 50-year-olds may have different maximum pulse rates, yet the individual with the lower max HR may be the stronger athlete. Discover the factors that determine an individual's heart rate response. In addition, endurance athletes quite often work too hard and never adequately develop their aerobic capacity. Understanding the appropriate heart rate zones will help you control the level of intensity of your workouts and therefore optimize your training growth. The zones of heart rate training are discussed, and they can be applied to all athletes.

Whether your goal is to improve your general health through walking, to incorporate cross-training into your fitness program, or to run your first 10K race, *Precision Heart Rate Training* has a wealth of information you can use. Heart rate training is not a gimmick—it tells the absolute truth about your fitness level. I hope you will enjoy new training opportunities through the simple method of monitoring your heart rate. Good luck!

Dave Scott
Five-Time Winner of the Ironman Triathlon

PREFACE

It was more than fifteen years ago that I was first introduced to wireless heart rate monitors and started using these miniature electronic devices with cyclists in preparation for the Los Angeles Olympic Games. Wireless heart rate monitors brought high-tech biofeedback training within the reach of all our athletes. All at once, heart rate monitors allowed our cyclists and coaches to develop sophisticated programs, which led to successful performances in competition.

This tradition continues today, with athletes and fitness enthusiasts using heart rate monitors to take the guesswork out of their training. The monitor serves as an excellent guide for those times when you need to accurately evaluate your performance and adjust your training regime. In many ways, training and competing with a heart rate monitor is like having a portable, full-time coach attached to your body.

Why is heart rate monitoring important? Your heart is the most important muscle in your body. In fact, it serves as a barometer for the rest of your body, telling you how hard you are exercising, how fast you are using up energy, and even what the state of your emotions is. It pulls these physiological variables together, weighs them, and then comes out with a single number that reports your overall condition.

Factors such as temperature, wind, humidity, altitude, terrain, and fitness levels can vary from workout to workout and affect the intensity of your effort. In the last few years, the heart rate monitor has allowed the exerciser to measure intensity by monitoring a key physiological response: heart rate. A heart rate monitor gives you this information immediately—while you're training or competing, or for that matter just out walking for health and fitness.

Over the last 15 years, the authors of this book have had the opportunity to introduce the benefits of heart rate monitoring to thousands of beginning athletes and elite athletes, in workshops and through the columns they write for several sport and fitness publications. In this book they explain and demonstrate to you the many uses of wireless heart rate monitoring for training and fitness evaluation. This book will also show you how to use a heart rate monitor to improve performance and how to obtain optimum results while exercising.

This book is written for those health and fitness enthusiasts, athletes, and coaches the authors cannot reach in person. It includes a full range of the authors' lectures, writings, and thoughts, as well as the workouts they recommend to the individuals they teach and coach. It teaches how the body can be trained to function at its best. It contains virtually all the scientific and practical facts athletes need to know about heart rate training and monitors. It is the most current, definitive, and practical book on heart rate training.

A heart rate monitor is a total performance-monitoring tool for the elite athlete as well as the fitness enthusiast. It may be the most important piece of fitness equipment you could own. The heart rate monitor has the potential to revolutionize training for health, fitness, and competition.

Best of luck,
Edmund R. Burke

ACKNOWLEDGMENTS

I would like to thank all the athletes, fitness enthusiasts, and others who, by their questions, have encouraged the authors to expand our knowledge of the relationships between heart rate monitoring and exercise. Those who have approached us have helped us realize the need for a book that explains the use of heart rate monitoring.

I would also like to thank the authors for contributing the excellent chapters found in this book. Their knowledge and dedication to improving the knowledge base of heart rate training have helped many people achieve their goals in athletics and fitness.

A big thank you to all the people at Polar CIC for their support in making this book a success. Polar has always been dedicated to educating the public about the benefits of heart rate monitoring for improved performance or a healthier lifestyle. Many more companies should follow their lead and put money into educating people about fitness and health.

To Human Kinetics and the support of Ted Miller to push this book through the corporate structure and onto the shelf. To Marni Basic, my editor, who once again has worked behind the scenes to make sure all the authors are proud of this book.

I am also grateful to the University of Colorado at Colorado Springs for the continued support they give me in my teaching, research, and writing, and for the opportunity to speak at many workshops and seminars around the world.

Finally, I want to thank my wife, Kathleen, who continues to put up with my strange and long hours at the computer, a busy travel schedule, my renewed life of training, and my verbal expressions, "I'm almost finished," and "I'll be back in a few hours from my bike ride."

CHAPTER 1

HEART RATE MONITORING AND TRAINING

EDMUND R. BURKE

All athletes, from beginners to Olympians, can benefit from using a heart rate monitor in training and competition. In many ways, training with a monitor is like having a full-time coach. For the athlete, a heart rate monitor can take the guesswork out of training intensity and also serve as an excellent motivator for those days when you want to accurately evaluate your performance and adjust your training regimen.

A monitor has been a staple for mountain bike champion Juli Furtado from Durango, Colorado. "If you are doing threshold work on the trails, it gives you an accurate reading of the intensity without having to guess at how hard the effort is," the Grundig champion said. "Instead of just saying you went really hard, you know when you are going hard. The monitor tells you."

Heart rate monitors will help the novice hold back and gradually build fitness. Conditioned athletes can use a monitor to hold back and keep their training within normal limits. Jim Campbell, medal winner in the World Master's Championships in the biathlon, not only uses a monitor for interval work but also puts one on for easy training days. "I know just how hard to run or cycle on easy days, and the monitor holds me back and allows me to recover from previous hard workouts," he says.

During races, a heart rate monitor can be used to determine whether you are going into anaerobic debt or pushing yourself too hard in hot weather. For example, several years ago Ingrid Kristiansen used her monitor in a 10K race when she wanted to break 33 minutes. Because of the environmental conditions that day the heat load on her body was great, and her monitor alerted her to the fact that she could not hold record pace under these environmental conditions. She was able to adjust her pace and win the race while saving herself from "blowing up" in the last few miles.

Kenny Souza, world-class duathlete from Boulder, Colorado, "uses his monitor all the time." Souza has said, "The monitor is also a good indicator for when I've overtrained. If I go out on a ride and know for a standard workout I cannot get my heart rate up to a predetermined level, I know it is time to back off. By the same token, if I can push my heart rate up to a high level consistently without feeling much of a lactate buildup in my legs, then I know my training is going well."

The Future Is Here

By providing positive feedback of workout parameters, a heart rate monitor serves as your "electronic coach." The monitor informs you of your state of fitness and enables you to see where improvement is needed in your training program to increase fitness. This is important in order for you to achieve maximum benefit from your training sessions without the risk of overworking. Used intelligently, a heart rate monitor will help you achieve your best performances.

Any fitness enthusiast, from the casual cyclist or runner to the dedicated master's athlete training for the Ironman Triathlon, can use a heart rate monitor for more efficient workouts. Likewise, many professional athletes have used heart rate monitors to better their performance.

Exercise not only should be based on the distance traveled, the amount of time involved, or the physical load; it should also be controlled by the degree of physical effort as measured by physiological signs. The American College of Sports Medicine

(ACSM), the world's leading medical and scientific authority on sports medicine and fitness, also emphasizes the need to measure heart rate as a tool for monitoring exercise intensity. In its position stand on the quality and quantity of fitness, the ACSM recommends that heart rate be monitored during exercise to determine the appropriate amount of exertion for the individual.

Heart rate informs you of the many changes taking place in your body while you are exercising. It tells you how hard you are exercising, whether your body is dehydrating too rapidly, whether you have recovered enough between intervals, or how fast you are using up energy. It is also a biofeedback tool.

Research conducted by Dr. James Rippe, Tufts University School of Medicine, published in 1995 in *Medicine, Exercise, Nutrition and Health,* suggests that simply watching your heart rate for about 10 minutes can be like meditation without the meditation. To put this idea to the test, researchers rounded up 55 women with high anxiety levels. For 10 minutes a day, 22 of the women snapped heart rate monitors (the kind used during exercise) around their torsos and watched their heart rates on the wristwatch that is part of the monitor. They saw immediate dips in daily anxiety as well as long-term changes in their anxiety. Twelve weeks later, these women had significantly reduced anxiety, depression, anger, and fatigue. The 34 women who spent their 10 minutes reading magazines had some changes in short-term anxiety but no big changes in how generally anxious they were.

The heart rate monitor is a very powerful tool for evaluating your training and health. It pulls together many physiological variables, weighs them, and comes up with a signal that reports your overall condition—heart rate.

How Heart Rate Monitors Work

The most critical feature of a heart monitor is its method of heart rate detection. The unreliable monitors attempt to detect heart rate at the earlobe or fingertip using inaccurate photo-optic techniques. Unfortunately, pulse detectors of this type are very sensitive to body movement and do not give accurate readings during exercise.

Thanks to modern electronics, portable wireless heart rate monitors are available that can measure heart rate per minute in

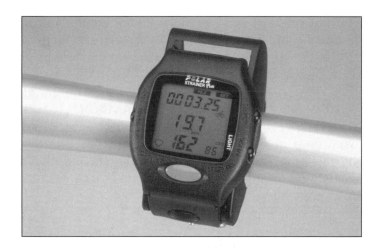

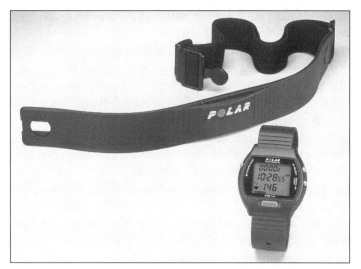

the field with the accuracy of expensive laboratory equipment. Currently, reliable wireless heart rate monitors employ electrocardiograph techniques that require a chest strap with rubber-covered electrodes and transmit heart rate to a wrist-worn or handlebar mount unit via telemetry. Several clinical studies published in the scientific literature showed that when an athlete was monitored both by a Polar heart rate monitor and a hardwired electrocardiograph unit, there was no significant difference between heart rate recordings.

Your training heart rate as displayed by the heart rate monitor measures your cardiovascular and physiological stress during your training session. Your training diary can now reflect an accurate level of intensity for a training session regardless of the speed you are riding at or the outside stresses on your body.

Why Monitoring Is So Important

The health of your heart is the most important reason to maintain fitness; fortunately, it is one of the easiest fitness goals to achieve. The heart is a muscle. The heart is always functioning, and therefore is maintaining itself; unfortunately, in many people the heart is operating at a relatively low level all day. But, as with any muscle, when periods of exercise are applied on a regular basis, the capacity of the heart will gradually increase so that it can deal with new tasks without strain. By monitoring your heart rate with a heart rate monitor, you can get more benefit out of the time spent exercising. As you may know, the three most important variables in designing a fitness program are frequency, duration, and intensity. The first two are easy to monitor, but the third can be elusive.

Fortunately, you have a built-in monitor that naturally gives you information on exercise intensity. It's your heart rate. It ranges from a minimum value when you're resting to a maximum level during hard exercise.

With the use of a heart rate monitor, you have at your disposal a powerful control tool for making your workouts more effective and time efficient, safer, and, equally important, much more fun. A heart rate monitor gives you a physiological window, through accurate heart rate measurement, into your body's response to the moment-to-moment changes in your physical activity.

Monitoring Physiological Variables

Now let's take a look at several cardiovascular physiological variables that are affected by training and by the environment that you will be exercising in while wearing a monitor.

Resting Heart Rate

At rest, your heart rate is regulated by signals from your brain that travel to your heart via the parasympathetic nervous system. The function of these nerves is to keep your heart beating regularly at a slow rate. Cardiovascular training increases the sensitivity of the heart to these nerves, which lowers the heart's resting rate even more. For example, some well-trained endurance athletes have resting heart rates as low as 30 to 50 beats per minute. The best time to measure resting heart rate is in the morning after waking up from a restful night of sleep. For several days, put on your heart rate monitor, lie in bed quietly for about five minutes, and record your heart rate. The average of five to seven days' recording can be used as your resting heart rate.

Although resting heart rate is generally lower in endurance athletes, it is not always a reliable indicator of aerobic fitness. For example, resting heart rate decreases with age and with some medications (especially a group of drugs called beta blockers, used to control high blood pressure and other cardiovascular diseases) and tends to increase with such factors as emotion, anticipation before exercise or a race, and the chemical stimulants caffeine and nicotine. Also, your heart rate should be measured in the same position, whether you are completely lying down or quietly sitting up in bed, since postural changes can affect the heart rate. Because of these factors, your fitness level could be falsely classified if you were to use resting heart rate alone as a measure of fitness.

However, monitored on a regular basis, a slower resting (morning) heart rate indicates increasing fitness. Conversely, a consistent increase in resting heart rate reflects overtraining or possibly dehydration, emotional stress, poor sleeping habits, illness, poor nutritional status, or a combination of two or more of these.

Heart Rate Response to Exercise

When you begin to exercise, the sympathetic nervous system and the adrenal glands located near the kidneys release a chemical messenger commonly called adrenaline, which stimulates the heart and increases your heart rate. Situations other than exercise may also activate this response. Anyone who has stood in front of a large group to give a presentation or has experienced intense turbulence on an airplane knows this quite well. If you took your pulse during these situations, you might find that your heart rate is actually in your "aerobic training zone" (or higher).

Why then doesn't an "activity" that causes an elevated heart rate, such as watching a suspenseful movie, lead to improved fitness? The answer is that during exercise, the increase in heart rate is directly related to the increase in oxygen delivered to the contracting skeletal muscles (increased oxygen consumption). It is the increase in oxygen consumption during exercise that is related to improving aerobic capacity (improved $\dot{V}O_2$max, or the maximum aerobic capacity at which the body can operate). Despite an increase in heart rate during psychological stress, the increase in oxygen consumption is only minimal because the muscles aren't utilizing oxygen to a great extent.

Your heart rate response to exercise actually changes as you become more aerobically fit. During any given submaximal exercise after three to six months of regular training, heart rate is reduced as much as 10 to 15 beats per minute as the result of cardiovascular conditioning. This means that if you started an exercise program of running at six miles per hour (one mile in 10 minutes) and your heart rate averaged 160 beats per minute, it would probably be only 145 beats per minute at the same pace after approximately eight weeks of running four to six days per week because of increased aerobic fitness. At that point you would have to start running harder to achieve the same desired training heart rate and to further improve your aerobic fitness. Once you have achieved your desired fitness level, however, no further increase in the intensity (training heart rate or exercise pace) is necessary to maintain that fitness.

Exercise Heart Rate: A Reflection of Metabolic Demand

As many people know from monitoring heart rate while exercising, it is obvious that the exercise heart rate is a reflection of overall physical exertion. But it is easy to forget that heart rate per se is not the variable of interest. Otherwise, as you have seen, you could drink half a dozen cups of coffee or ride a roller coaster and watch your cardiovascular fitness improve. Heart rate is a valid measure of exercise

→

intensity only if it reflects metabolic rate, which can be measured by oxygen consumption, or $\dot{V}O_2$. In fact, exercise oxygen consumption would be the best measure of metabolic rate during exercise, but we have no convenient way to measure this variable outside of the laboratory. Fortunately, there is a relatively linear relationship between oxygen consumption and heart rate during exercise, so we use exercise heart rate to estimate exercise metabolic rate.

Table 1.1 shows the relationship between relative heart rate and percentage of maximal oxygen consumption ($\dot{V}O_2$max). This chart is a reminder that an exercise heart rate representing 50 percent of maximal heart rate (MHR) does not mean a person is working at 50 percent of his or her working capacity.

TABLE 1.1	Relationship Between Relative Heart Rate and $\dot{V}O_2$max	
Percent MHR		**Percent $\dot{V}O_2$ max**
35		30
60		50
80		75
90		84
100		100

Maximal Heart Rate

One of the first things people must do in using a heart rate monitor is to determine their MHR. Your MHR (beats per minute) is the highest number of times your heart can contract in one minute. Once you know how fast your heart beats when you're exercising all out, you can figure your target heart rate zones—the percentages you must know in order to design a sensible training program.

It also appears that for the most part, MHR is determined by genetics and age. In addition, it does not vary much. After age 20 or so, MHR in sedentary individuals begins to decrease about one beat per year; but generally speaking, if you train fairly hard, your MHR will stay about the same over the years. It certainly does not rise or fall with your level of fitness as much as resting and submaximal heart rates do.

Before you can determine the optimal heart rate limits that will enable you to train for competition or embark upon a fitness program most effectively, you should know your MHR. You can estimate MHR from the following formula:

$$MHR = 220 - age\ (in\ years).$$

This means that the mean MHR for a 40-year-old male will be 220 – 40 = 180 beats per minute.

You should nevertheless bear in mind that actual MHRs can vary individually by as many as 15 beats without implying the presence of any illness (more on this in chapter 2).

If you are new to sport, are returning after a lengthy break, or have a history of heart disease, this simple formula will suffice and is recommended by the American Heart Association and the ACSM for determining heart rate. Because it is an "average," it is not very accurate, especially for individuals who are very fit or who want to determine their MHR.

The most accurate way to determine your MHR is to have it clinically tested (usually on a treadmill or bicycle ergometer) by a physician or clinician trained in maximal stress testing. Or you could use time trials under the supervision of a trained coach or exercise physiologist.

In any case, determining your actual MHR is the key to constructing a well-designed heart rate monitor training program. How do you do that?

While it is often recommended that people complete a treadmill or stationary bicycle test to determine their MHR, in the chapters on individual sports you will be given suggested tests for determining your true MHR in that particular activity.

A word of caution and advice: Do not take these self-administered field tests if you are over the age of 35, have a history of heart disease in your family, are overweight, have been sedentary for a number of years, or are in poor physical condition. The ACSM also suggests that among those who are symptom free and in whom no major risk factors are present, women over the age of 50 and men over the age of 40 should have physician supervision when completing a maximal test.

The lack of precision of the 220 minus age formula can also lead to poor training for the serious athlete. Take the case of a 42-year-old female marathon runner who thinks her MHR is 178 beats per minute and wants to work out at 80 percent of MHR (which is also about 75 percent of $\dot{V}O_2$max—a frequently recommended training intensity). She runs along with a heart rate of 142 beats per minute (80 percent of 178) during her training runs, but—unknown to her—her MHR is really 195 beats per minute, and therefore her training heart rate of 142 is only 73 percent of maximal, not 80 percent. She should be attaining a heart rate of 156 beats per minute during her workout. In general, if you use the 220 minus age formula to plan the intensity of your workouts and your actual MHR falls below the 220 minus age prediction, you'll tend to run too quickly during your training sessions; if your MHR is higher than predicted, you'll run too slowly.

We will have more discussion on estimating your MHR in chapter 2.

Maximal Heart Rate Is Sport Specific

Not all exercises cause the same MHR response. Heart rate response can be affected by variables such as body posture and the size of the muscle mass involved in the exercise. As a general rule, the bigger the muscle masses involved during exercise, the higher the MHR and $\dot{V}O_2$max. For instance, MHR is about 10–13 beats per minute (5–6 percent) lower in freestyle swimming as compared to running by both trained and untrained individuals. This can be explained by the important contribution of the arms as opposed to the legs in swimming and by the horizontal position of the body, which facilitates venous return to the heart. In the case of swimming, the water may also produce a cooling effect on the body. In other forms of arm exercise, such as arm pedaling, MHR values of 170–180 beats per minute are usually reported for able-bodied individuals and for people who are dependent on wheelchairs but are nonparaplegic.

Even when large muscle masses such as the legs are involved, MHR can vary according to the type of exercise performed. For instance, MHR tends to be lower during cycling than during

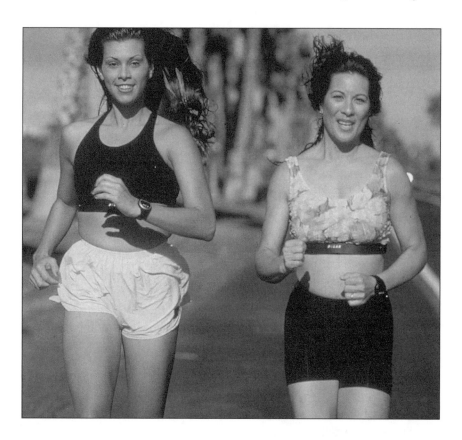

running. This could be explained by the fact that some blood is "trapped" in the legs during cycling exercise, thus decreasing venous return from the lower extremities and reducing stroke volume (the amount of blood pumped by the heart during each contraction).

For example, my MHR is 187 beats per minute for running, 180 beats per minute for cycling, and 175 beats per minute for swimming. The differences among these three activities are significant enough that I plan my training around the appropriate MHR.

Heart Rate During Submaximal Exercise

Heart rate during submaximal exercise can be affected by a wide variety of factors that you need to consider when designing training programs or monitoring your training intensities during exercise. Knowing these factors will give you a better understanding of the relationship between heart rate and workload.

Effect of Muscle Mass Involved

At submaximal intensities, the pattern of the heart rate-$\dot{V}O_2$ relationship is affected by the muscle mass involved in the exercise. As figure 1.1 shows, during exercise involving large muscle mass (e.g., the legs in cycling or running), heart rate at a given submaximal workload is lower than when smaller muscle masses are involved (e.g., when the arms are used in arm cycling).

Aerobic activities that include significant upper-body movements, and aerobics with the concomitant use of hand weights, may elicit heart rates 10 to 15 beats per minute higher than the heart rates for running or cycling at the same percentage of aerobic capacity. This could be explained by a reduced stroke volume and a higher peripheral resistance to blood flow resulting from a constriction in the blood vessels of the inactive muscles. Static (isometric) exercise also increases the heart rate above the values

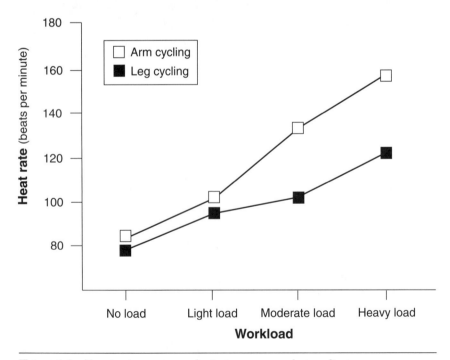

Figure 1.1   Heart rate response during arm versus leg cycling.

expected from the workload. You often see this when someone is lifting or pushing a heavy load.

Although the prescribed heart rate for arm training should ideally be based on the results of a progressive exercise test of the upper extremities, this may not always be feasible. Research indicates that a slightly lower MHR is typically obtained during arm-exercise than during leg-exercise testing. As a result, an arm-exercise prescription based on an MHR obtained during leg ergometry may result in an inappropriately high target heart rate for upper-extremity training. As a general rule, the prescribed exercise heart rate for leg training should be reduced by approximately 10 beats per minute for arm training. In addition, you should monitor your rate of perceived exertion and use it as a secondary guide to know how hard you're exercising your heart.

In estimating the appropriate work rates for arm training, it is important to remember that although maximal physiologic responses are generally greater during leg exercise than during arm exercise, the heart rate, blood pressure, and oxygen uptake for arm exercise are higher for any given submaximal work rate. As a result, an exercise work rate considered appropriate for leg training will be too high for arm training. A work rate approximating 50 percent of that used for leg training is, generally, appropriate for arm training. For example, if you exercise at 150 watts for leg training, you should train at 75 watts for arm training. Even though the work rate for the arms is considerably lower than the power output for the legs, the heart rates and the ratings of perceived exertion would generally be comparable.

Effect of Psychological Stress

Stress and other emotions can affect heart response both before and during exercise. Have you ever observed your heart rate prior to a 100-meter sprint? The elevated preexercise heart rate can be attributed to the high level of anticipation before this type of event. Measured heart rates just before the start of competitions of various lengths, studied by McArdle and others from Queens University in New York, show that heart rates are lower in longer races—approximately 130, 120, and 110 beats per minute, respectively, for the 400-, 800-, and 3,000-meter events.

In 1986, Åstrand and Rodhal, researchers from Sweden, evaluated a world-class skier's heart rate during a competition. Heart rate for the skier at the start of the event was 160 beats per minute; it reached a maximum of 207 beats per minute toward the end of the race. However, when the same course was run on a subsequent day in training, heart rate values were much lower and the actual intensity was estimated at approximately 80 percent of the skier's $\dot{V}O_2$max.

These data show that heart rate is not always a good indicator of the physical demands of an activity, particularly when the performer is anxious or under stress. At low to moderate workloads, this can result in a significant overestimation of work intensity. However, the effect of psychological stress on heart rate response will become less important as the exercise gets near maximum effort. It may be wise to use your heart rate monitor in competition in order to find out how your heart rate responds to competition and whether you can adequately control your emotions.

Effect of Heat, Clothing, and Cold

In response to the elevation in body temperature that results from exercise, surface cooling is enhanced as blood is diverted to the skin and sweating rate is increased. At the same time, an adequate blood flow to the working muscles must be maintained so that they are supplied with oxygen and fuel, such as glucose and fats. Under these conditions, the body faces a circulatory challenge as the skin and the active muscles "compete" for blood. Heart rate may increase as much as 5 to 10 beats per minute over one hour of running or cycling at the same intensity (oxygen consumption) in moderate weather, and it may increase even more in hot and humid weather. This is often referred to as "cardiac drift" or "cardiac creep" (see page 77 for more information).

Also, as temperatures begin to drop below 50 degrees Fahrenheit (about 10 degrees Celsius), resting heart rate will increase in an individual who is lightly clothed. This is because the body will begin to release hormones that affect the muscles and heart so that they contract in order to increase metabolism to maintain the body's core temperature.

Look at figure 1.2 and notice the cardiac or heart rate increase. The athlete is not increasing speed while cycling, but the heart rate is being forced to increase to compensate for decreased stroke volume.

Clothing also has a significant effect on heart rate response both during and following exercise. Clothing insulates the body from its surroundings, which reduces its ability to dissipate heat generated by the working muscles. This phenomenon is further accentuated by impermeable-type clothing. In conditions in which insulation is moderate, successive work intervals result in a higher heart rate despite adequate recovery time.

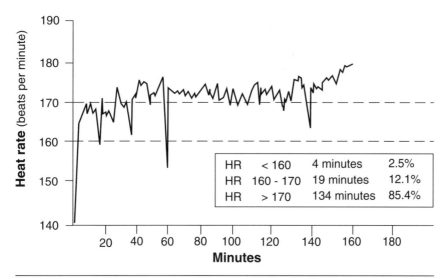

Figure 1.2 Cardiac drift during a 170-minute bike ride. Athlete rode at same speed throughout the duration of the ride.

Analysis of your heart rate recorded during exercise must take into account the circulatory adjustments described previously, particularly during exercise in a hot environment. If not, the absolute work intensity at which you have performed will be overestimated. Heart rate will tend to be higher toward the end of prolonged exercise as a result of dehydration and increased body temperature, even though the actual intensity remains constant. Clothing and/or protective equipment will result in higher heart rates during submaximal exercise and recovery.

Effect of Altitude

At any given submaximal workload, heart rate will be higher for exercise at altitude as compared to sea level. At altitude, when you perform an exercise session at a given percentage of MHR, you will be exercising (working) at an absolute lower workload. Since your blood cells are carrying less oxygen, your heart beats more often to compensate for the lower oxygen carried by the red blood cells. When heart rate at a given absolute intensity returns to near sea-level values, it is a sign that you have acclimatized to the altitude. Your body has increased its number of red blood cells to help carry more oxygen. However, because of the lower air density at altitude, your response may vary if air represents smaller resistance factor, such as in speed skating or cycling.

Day-to-Day Variation in Heart Rate

Even when you try to standardize conditions from workout to workout, day-to-day variations of up to plus or minus five beats per minute can be observed at the same submaximal workloads. This could be due to chronic dehydration, changes in circulating hormone levels, glycogen depletion, or lack of full recovery from the previous day's training or racing.

Effect of Gender

On the average, the MHR of well-trained females is slightly lower than or similar to that of males of the same age group. However, women

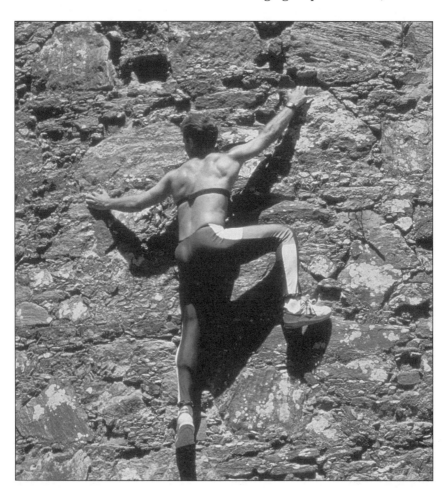

generally have a higher heart rate response than men to the same absolute submaximal workload. Heart rate recovery is also generally slower in females than in males. The differences between males and females are most likely explained by the generally smaller dimensions of the female heart, which results in lower stroke volume. Consequently, the female heart has to beat more often to achieve a particular cardiac output.

Effect of Exercise in Water

More and more athletes and fitness enthusiasts are turning to water-based exercise programs for cross-training or for continuation of training during recovery from injury. A person can perform aerobics, walking, and running in the water either while standing in chest-deep water or while using a buoyancy vest in deeper water.

In water, you are virtually weightless. The buoyancy of water effectively supports 90 percent of the body's weight. Consequently, when you exercise in water you are moving only 10 percent of your weight. When suspended with a flotation belt, you're able to move in ways not possible on land. This suspended position in water decreases stress on joints, enabling greater freedom of movement.

In water there is resistance in all directions. The density of water is 12 times greater than that of air, creating a balanced resistance that is equal on all sides. In water you choose the intensity of your workout because the water's resistance is determined by the speed of your movements. To maximize resistance, you can increase speed and enlarge the surface area that is moved through the water (e.g., by cupping the hands, pointing the toes, or using resistive equipment).

The unique properties of water enable your heart to work more efficiently. The hydrostatic pressure of the water pushes equally on all body surfaces and acts as an auxiliary heart pump, reducing the number of heartbeats per minute. Consequently, your heart rate is an estimated 10–13 beats lower per minute during suspended water exercise than for the same effort on land. This means you are getting the same training effect with fewer beats per minute. In addition, the temperature of the water will often reduce the heat buildup, allowing the circulatory system to concentrate on getting blood to the muscles instead of to the skin for cooling.

As an estimate, add 10 percent to your in-water heart rate to get an idea of what the on-land heart rate would be. For example, if your heart rate is 130 in water, add 13, for the equivalent of 143 on land.

Using Heart Rate and Ratings of Perceived Exertion to Monitor Exercise Intensity

Another method for prescribing and monitoring exercise intensity involves the use of ratings of perceived exertion (RPE). Perceived exertion refers to the physical strain an individual believes he or she is experiencing while exercising. Perceived-exertion feedback is important because it provides a practical means for individuals to become sensitive to what constitutes appropriate exercise intensity. During exercise, perception of effort is influenced by a variety of cues—some local in nature (e.g., sensations of muscular discomfort or strain) and some central in nature (e.g., heart rate, breathing rate, etc.).

The most common measurement tool for assessing perceived exertion is a rating scale named after its developer, Swedish psychologist Gunnar Borg. Borg's pioneering concepts relating to perceived exertion have evolved dramatically over the years. Originally, Borg proposed a scale (also referred to as the RPE Scale) that utilized 15 stages (numbered from 6 to 20) of sensations, 7 of which were identified by descriptors (refer to table 1.2, which shows 5 of these descriptors).

Borg's original efforts were based on the premise that his numbering system closely correlated to heart rate. When a zero was added to each category number, a range of numbers comparable to the heart rate range in young, trained individuals (60 to 200 beats per minute) was created. Borg's initial RPE Scale followed the patterns of heart rate and oxygen consumption during incremental aerobic exercise. As exercise intensity increased, heart rate, oxygen consumption, and RPE increased.

For example, an RPE of 7 would approximate a heart rate of 70 beats per minute; an RPE of 14 would approximate a heart rate of 140. The RPE response correlates well with cardiovascular and metabolic factors such as heart rate, breathing, oxygen consumption, and overall fatigue.

Perhaps the most appropriate use of the RPE Scale is as a supplement to heart rate monitoring. An example of an appropriate time to use both heart rate and RPE is with an individual who is at high risk and is just beginning an exercise program. People in this situation should monitor with both methods to ensure close observation of their physiological and cardiac response to the exercise session.

Recently, Rod Dishman, PhD, a researcher from the University of Georgia, has suggested an alternative approach to the RPE Scale because he believes that it is somewhat prone to error in individuals who have not received proper instructions and guidance in its use during exercise. His alternative approach is termed "Preferred Exertion." Using Preferred Exertion allows people to self-select their exercise intensity or power output according to their own volition, as long as the intensity stays within an effective target zone such as the ACSM's suggested 60 to 90 percent of MHR.

Research is now being fostered to see whether "Preferred Exertion" better promotes long-term exercise adherence in conjunction with a properly prescribed exercise heart rate intensity. Many researchers feel that being observant of perceptual and intensity indicators such as RPE and Preferred Exertion may be beneficial especially if one is using a target heart rate zone based on a predicted MHR.

TABLE 1.2 Classification of Exercise Intensity and Ratings of Perceived Exertion

Percent MHR	Heart Rate reserve or percent of $\dot{V}O_2$ max	Rating of perceived exertion	Classification of intensity
< 35	< 30	< 9	Very light
35–59	30–49	10–11	Light
60–79	50–74	12–13	Moderate
80–89	75–84	14–16	Heavy
> 90	> 85	> 16	Very heavy

Using Submaximal Heart Rates to Monitor Overtraining and Illness

Heart rate is a good indicator of how recovered you are from a hard workout or race. Occasionally, sleep with your heart monitor on and compare your morning heart rate for successive days. "Your mind may say you are rested, but your heart rate may actually be elevated upon waking," cautions Skip Hamilton, coach to several top-ranked off-road cyclists and senior coach at the Davis Phinney-Connie Carpenter training camps. "This is a sign that your body is not fully rested and something is amiss. This is not a time to take on any hard training."

You can also test your recovery during training. You can use your heart rate with perceived exertion, the feeling of effort. By using a heart rate monitor you learn to associate what specific intensities or paces feel like, and you can use this in training and racing to guide your performances.

Or you can use a heart rate monitor to signal overtraining or lack of recovery. For example, during an interval session, your heart rate during a standard effort should be 170–180 beats per minute and the effort should feel hard. If you are not recovered, the same level of perceived exertion may correspond to a heart rate of, let's say, 150–160 beats per minute. "This is a good sign that you are not ready to take on a hard training session. Sometimes I see this happen when an athlete has just had an excellent weekend of racing and feels good. But during the next hard session if his heart rate is lower for the same perceived effort, I tell him to take an easy day," says Hamilton. "Heart rate is a true barometer to how recovered you are and when you can take on more training."

"The monitor is a good indicator for when you've overtrained," says Andy Hampsten, previous winner of l'Alpe d'Huez, one of the toughest stages of the Tour de France. "If I go out on a ride and know for a standard workout I cannot get my heart rate up to a predetermined level, I know it is time to back off. By the same token, if I can push my heart rate up to a high level consistently without feeling much of a lactic acid buildup in my legs, then I know my training is going well." A heart rate monitor helps prevent under- or overexertion.

Heart rate can also help you come back from illness. "After coming back from an illness or injury you are usually putting out a minimal work output, but your heart rate may be reading high during these efforts," states Hamilton. "You cannot know this without a heart rate monitor. Back off the pace for a few days until they match; that is, your heart rate is back to the perceived level of exertion of effort when you are healthy."

Using Heart Rate to Monitor Anaerobic/Lactate Threshold

What does anaerobic threshold (AT) mean? At lower training intensities, our metabolism has no trouble supplying enough energy by burning glucose and/or fat in the presence of oxygen. At high intensities, our heart, lungs, and circulatory system cannot supply enough oxygen to keep up with demand. Our body compensates by burning glucose in a short-term chemical reaction that does not require oxygen (anaerobic means "without oxygen").

The problem with anaerobic energy production is that it is good for only a few seconds before waste products like lactic acid rapidly build up. Have you ever tried to sprint for longer than 90 seconds? You will know what I am talking about!

Athletes refer to the intensity at which we begin to "go anaerobic" and build up lactic acid as our AT. I should mention that the terms "anaerobic threshold" and "lactate threshold" are often used interchangeably by athletes, even though you will hear the scientific community refer to it as the lactate threshold.

It is useful to train for short periods (three to five minutes) at a heart rate just below this point because your AT heart rate increases as you get fit.

You should reserve this hard-intensity training for

1. times when you have been training for some months and are confident of your fitness,
2. times when you have competitive aspirations,
3. exercise in short, sharp bursts of 3 to 5 minutes' duration (interval training) for many athletes (highly trained and

experienced athletes can increase these efforts to 10 to 20 minutes at this intensity), and

4. racing (most athletes can maintain this intensity for about one hour).

Originally, it was thought that AT was an exact heart rate beyond which lactic acid suddenly started to accumulate. Modern research tells us that it is not a sudden, easily marked point, but a more gradual transition.

It remains a useful idea, though. When we are unfit, our AT might be at 65 to 70 percent effort or lower. As our training progresses, our AT shifts upward such that in a very fit competitive athlete it might be at 85 to 90 percent effort. Simply put, an unfit person may be able to hold only 70 percent effort for one hour, while a very fit athlete may be able to hold 90 percent effort!

For most activities, this hard training is best reserved for one session per week, and maybe two, but only if the person is reasonably fit. Swimming is a little different. Because the body is suspended in water, two or three AT sessions per week does not seem to pose a problem.

You can make a very good guess of your own AT by the following methods:

1. One-hour time trial. We can maintain our AT heart rate for about one hour. Record your heart rate for best effort and average it for the hour.

2. Gradually speeding up over at least 10 minutes while cycling or running. As you reach your AT heart rate, your legs will begin to feel a little like rubber and suddenly your rate of breathing will increase. This is not because you need more oxygen but because the extra acid in the blood speeds up the breathing control center in your brain. Glance at your monitor and take note of your heart rate. This can be a very accurate method.

3. The chapters that follow will give you more specific ways to determine your AT for a particular sport or activity.

Using Heart Rate and Lactate

With the advent of automated lactate analyzers in the early 1980s, it became much easier to obtain lactic acid measurements quickly and accurately. Recently, portable analyzers have arrived on the market, making immediate measurement possible at the competition or training site. Now this useful training tool is within the reach of small colleges and athletic clubs where sophisticated laboratories, trained exercise scientists, and complex testing methods are unavailable.

Simultaneous heart rate and lactate measurements enable a person to tell whether he or she is exercising aerobically or anaerobically as measured by heart rate. Depending on the lactate, the heart rate can be adjusted up or down to maintain a specific lactate level during training. Thus, if the lactate values are too high for the particular endurance workload, that is, above 4 millimoles per liter (mmol/L), the heart rate during training can be adjusted downward. If the lactate is too low, that is, under 1.5 mmol/L, the heart rate during training can be increased. It is then possible to check the workload on the basis of the training heart rate determined for this particular individual from the lactate levels. During training, heart rate should be checked by lactate measurements about every four weeks. The heart rate during exercise can thus be individually tailored, optimizing the exertion level and achieving effective training.

The following examples show the advantages of this two-pronged (heart rate and lactate) check on exercise intensity: figure 1.3 shows the record of a 20-year-old middle-distance runner's heart rate during a 30-minute run. The average rate is about 165 beats per minute. The lactate concentration was monitored at three times during the run, and on each occasion it was about 3 mmol/L, confirming that this was the correct workload for an individual during endurance training or jogging for health. Usually, a value of 4 mmol/L or lower is good for persons interested in aerobic conditioning.

Figure 1.4 also shows good agreement between the heart rate and the corresponding lactate level. The heart rate of runner A (50 years old) increased during exercise to about 120 beats per minute, somewhat below a heart rate of 120 to 136 beats per minute (a heart rate zone of 70 percent to 80 percent), an intensity good for aerobic conditioning. The

→

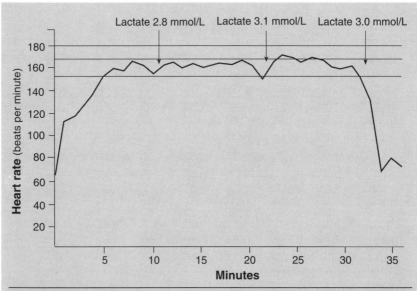

Figure 1.3 Heart rate and lactate during a 30-minute run by a 20-year-old middle-distance runner.

lactic acid level remained at 2 mmol/L throughout the run. Runner B (aged 49) exercised at approximately the same heart rate, clearly above his lactate threshold, and had a corresponding increase in lactate, at one time to 6 mmol/L.

In practice, clear deviations in lactate production can occur from exercising at a predetermined exercise intensity. For example, let's look at the effects of using an estimated threshold intensity of 85 percent of MHR for two well-trained runners, which would be a good estimate of lactate threshold in a highly trained individual. Although runner C (40 years old) in figure 1.5 exercised at approximately 85 percent of his MHR (153 beats per minute), his lactate concentration rose to 6 mmol/L, which may be too high an intensity since his lactate continued to rise during the run, reaching 8 mmol/L at the end of the run. Runner D, the same age, exercised at the same estimated threshold of 85 percent of MHR heart rate (again 150 to 153 beats per minute), but if one considers his lactate, which rose to just under 4 mmol/L and leveled off during the run, the workload was chosen correctly. These examples show how one can use a lactate analyzer with a heart rate monitor to control exercise intensity.

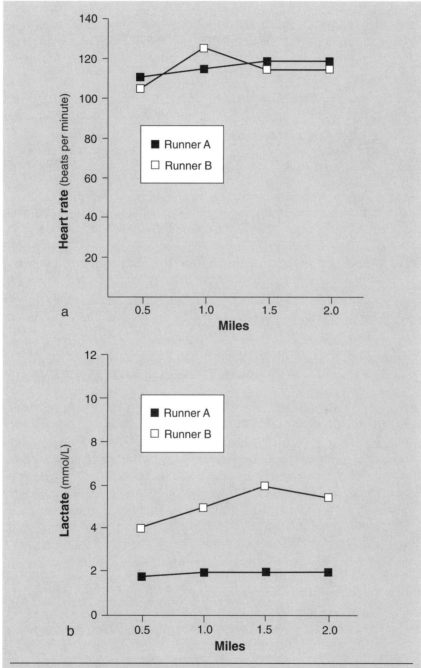

Figure 1.4   Heart rate (a) and lactate (b) for two runners during a two-mile run.

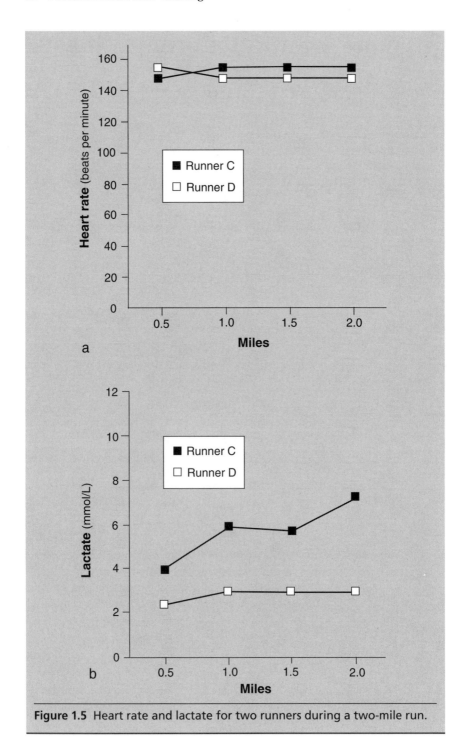

Figure 1.5 Heart rate and lactate for two runners during a two-mile run.

Training With a Heart Rate Monitor

The value of using heart rate as a tool in exercise programs has been understood for a long time. It just hasn't always been an easy tool to use.

Exercise physiologists, fitness enthusiasts, and athletes used to have a tough time getting a quick and accurate reading while they were moving vigorously. The best way seemed to be to stop exercising long enough to take a pulse reading and then start up again.

You could always take the pulse more easily after a bout of exercise, so measuring recovery heart rate became popular. Even the best exercise physiology laboratories, with their very expensive metabolic carts, had their share of problems recording exercise heart rate while subjects panted and thrashed on treadmills and bicycle ergometers.

But their diligence paid off. Some of the secrets of achieving aerobic fitness were revealed and, not surprisingly, were keyed to specific levels of heart rate. The public learned about age-related target zones and about both aerobic and anaerobic thresholds in the mid-1970s. But the popularity of heart rate training still suffered from the inconvenience of using it.

Now those days are gone. Today's heart rate monitors are light, accurate, affordable, and painless to use.

Heart rate monitors as training aids can be used in several important ways to make your training sessions more effective. They allow you to design effective training programs using the concept of target heart rate "zone" training. The exercise heart rate "target zone" is the range of effort that will give you a good training effect. In the next chapter, you will learn how to design target heart rate zones to optimize your training and competition.

CHAPTER 2

BETTER TRAINING WITH HEART RATE ZONES

EDMUND R. BURKE

Probably the most exciting aspect of having the ability to immediately and constantly know your heart rate is that it allows for "zone" training. This type of training allows you to train within certain heart rate zones to achieve the desired goals of specific workouts.

Since heart rate is related to oxygen consumption during exercise, you can simply measure your heart rate to get a good indication of your exercise intensity. In 1994 the American College of Sports Medicine published its position stand on the quality and quantity of exercise, recommending that the intensity of training necessary to improve or maintain cardiorespiratory fitness is in the range of 50 to 85 percent of maximal aerobic capacity, or $\dot{V}O_2$max. This corresponds to a range of 65 to 90 percent of your maximal heart rate (MHR). Your MHR is the highest heart rate you achieve in an all-out effort to the point of exhaustion. For many individuals, pushing to this level may not be desirable or safe. An approximation of MHR can be made instead by using the simple formula 220 minus your age. But, as stated in the last chapter, you should try to complete a sports-specific or laboratory maximal stress test to determine your true MHR.

Establishing Target Heart Rates

The target heart rate is established using a percentage of your MHR. For example, the following calculation of target heart rate (THR) is for a 35-year-old person using a moderate training range of 70 to 80 percent of age-predicted MHR:

$$MHR = 220 - 35 = 185 \text{ beats per minute.}$$
$$THR = 185 \times .70 = 130 \text{ beats per minute.}$$
$$THR = 185 \times .80 = 148 \text{ beats per minute.}$$

This method can be used to estimate your aerobic training zone. Another method you can employ is called the heart rate reserve method or Karvonen method, which uses the difference between true MHR (as measured in laboratory or field stress test) and resting heart rate (RHR).

$$\text{Target heart rate reserve (THHR)} =$$
$$[(MHR - RHR) \times \% \text{ exercise intensity}] + RHR.$$
$$\text{THHR for 70 percent} = [(MHR - RHR) \times .70] + RHR.$$
$$\text{THHR for 80 percent} = [(MHR - RHR) \times .80] + RHR.$$

An example of this method, also using 70 to 80 percent intensity for a 35-year-old who has a true MHR of 183 beats per minute and a resting heart rate of 65 beats per minute, is as follows:

$$[(183 - 65) \times .70] + 65 = 148 \text{ beats per minute.}$$
$$[(183 - 65) \times .80] + 65 = 159 \text{ beats per minute.}$$

Notice that the target heart rate (beats per minute) is higher using the heart rate reserve (HRR) method. This is so because the HRR method more closely indicates actual $\dot{V}O_2$ than does a set percentage of MHR. Refer back to table 1.2. Target heart rate using 80 percent of the MHR, for example, is only 75 percent of $\dot{V}O_2$max, whereas 80 percent with the HRR method is closer to 80 percent of

$\dot{V}O_2$max. It is important to realize, however, that there are no strong scientific data to support the advantage of one method over the other, since they are equally effective in establishing training thresholds.

Whatever method is used, it is always in a beginner's best interest to start at the low end of the range and progress to the upper end of the range. Also, health benefits of exercise such as a reduced risk of developing heart disease can be attained with regular physical activity that is performed well below the minimal threshold needed to improve aerobic fitness.

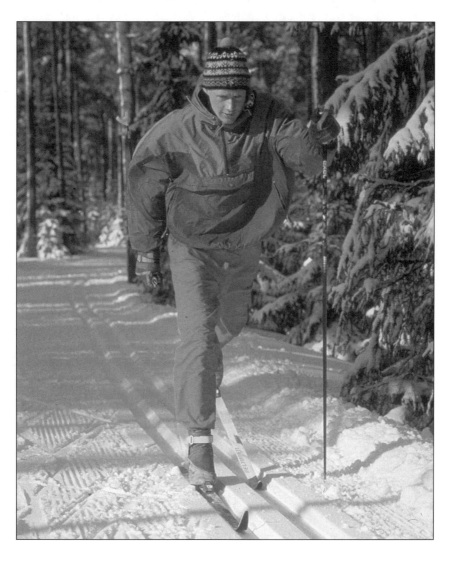

Current Research on Using Heart Rate Reserve

Most books about exercise training state that the HRR method of prescribing target heart rates provides the same exercise intensity as the equivalent percentage of $\dot{V}O_2$max. For example, if you are at 70 percent of HRR, you are supposedly at 70 percent of $\dot{V}O_2$max. However, HRR is a measure of *net* heart rate—how much your heart rate during exercise is above the resting value. Theoretically, it should relate directly to the net oxygen consumption, the increase above rest, rather than the gross oxygen consumption, expressed as a percentage of $\dot{V}O_2$max. Recently researchers at Old Dominion University examined the discrepancy between these percentages (%HRR and %$\dot{V}O_2$max) and then compared %HRR to the percentage of $\dot{V}O_2$ reserve—a term for the net oxygen consumption.[1]

For the study, 63 subjects exercised on a laboratory bicycle while oxygen consumption and heart rate were measured. The subjects pedaled at a constant 80 revolutions per minute while the resistance was increased every three minutes. This continued until the work was so severe that the subjects were unable to keep pedaling. Heart rates measured at the end of every three minutes were expressed as percentages of HRR and then were compared to the oxygen consumption measured at the same time.

The researchers found that values of %HRR and %$\dot{V}O_2$max did not match up. The two sets of values were fairly close for very intense exercise, but the difference became increasingly greater for more moderate training levels, Then the researchers compared the %HRR values with the percentage of $\dot{V}O_2$ reserve (%$\dot{V}O_2$ reserve). $\dot{V}O_2$ reserve, like HRR, is calculated by subtracting the resting $\dot{V}O_2$ from the maximal $\dot{V}O_2$. Then, the net $\dot{V}O_2$ that is used during a given level of exercise is expressed as a percentage of that range. The researchers found that the values of %HRR and %$\dot{V}O_2$ reserve were almost identical. In fact, when the two sets of values were plotted against each other on a graph, the line drawn through the data had a slope of 1.00 and an intercept of –0.1; in other words, it rose exactly one %HRR unit for one %V̇O₂ reserve unit and passed almost exactly through the origin.

The researchers concluded that HRR is a nearly perfect indicator of V̇O₂ reserve. This makes it the best way to prescribe exercise intensity. An athlete simply decides what intensity level he or she wishes to train at: for example, 60 to 70 percent of net V̇O₂ for a moderate-intensity, longer-duration workout, or 80 to 90 percent for a short, hard-pace workout. The intensity percentage is then used in the calculation of target heart rate using the HRR formula:

THR = [(MHR − RHR) × (intensity percentage)] + RHR.

Note: [1] Swain, D.P. (1997, March) Heart rate reserve is equivalent to % V̇O₂ reserve, not V̇O₂ max. *Medicine and Science in Sports and Exercise.* 29: 410-414.

Errors in Estimating Maximal Heart Rate Using 220 Minus Your Age

Although 220 minus age is a rule of thumb, individual values vary plus or minus from this average value by approximately 15 beats per minute, as stated in the American College of Sports Medicine's *Guidelines for Exercise Testing and Prescription* (Lea & Febiger, 1991). To illustrate, using 220 minus age plus or minus 15 beats (15 as the standard deviation), we can see that a 40-year-old would have an estimated MHR of 180 beats per minute (220 – 40 = 180) but that most 40-year-olds would fall somewhere between 165 and 195 beats per minute (180 + or – 15 beats per minute). This shows the large potential error in estimating someone's MHR. Consequently, although it often appears that a person is either above or below his or her calculated target heart rate based on age-predicted MHR, that person may, in fact, be exercising in a training-sensitive zone that is both safe and effective for improving fitness.

The 220 minus age formula is based on the fact that MHR declines with age at the rate of about one beat per year. This is generally true for someone who has a sedentary lifestyle and does very little exercise.

Recent research reported by Kallio and Seppanen from Finland showed, however, that 205 minus 1/2 age is more accurate for predicting MHRs for people who are described as "chronically fit"—those who have slowed the aging process by staying in shape.

This discovery is important for masters and senior athletes. Take me as an example. At age 48 and having been fairly active my whole life, my MHR is 180—very close to the predicted value of 181 using the 205 minus 1/2 age formula, and 8 beats above the 172 predicted by 220 minus age equation. Those extra 8 beats help me better fit into the five target heart rate zones to be described in the next section. I would wind up undertrained if I did not realize that a lifetime of exercise has kept my heart "younger" than my legs.

But remember that both these formulas, as well as other published equations, are just predicting your MHR. If the numbers you generate in workouts don't make any sense when you plug them into the appropriate formulas in this book, you may need to do a sport-specific MHR test to determine your true MHR.

Another potential limitation with the use of heart rate to gauge training intensity is the possibility of error in measurement when you are trying to determine your heart rate by palpating your heart rate on your carotid artery (artery on the side of your neck) or on the back of your wrist. This error is particularly common for novice exercisers who probably would benefit the most from monitoring their heart rates during training. Studies conducted by Dr. Rippe of Tufts University, and at other research institutes, showed that when individuals tried to determine their heart rates by palpating their carotid arteries, they were often off by as much as 20 beats per minute when the 10-second count was taken out to 60 seconds.

The Four Training Zones

There are four general heart rate training zones of different levels of training intensity, each of which corresponds to various metabolic or respiratory transport mechanisms within your body. All of these zones can be tracked by your heart rate monitor.

The zones you see listed in this chapter are the most commonly quoted by coaches and athletes, but they are not the only way of describing training intensities. In later chapters of this book, you will be introduced to different training zones by the various authors. The key point to remember is that while the zone percentages may vary by chapter and the authors may use different training terminology, the objective is the same: to train your body's various energy systems with various heart rate zones.

In addition, some coaches and athletes choose training zones based on anaerobic threshold heart rate. For example, Dave Scott, past Ironman champion, uses anaerobic threshold heart rate as the basis of his training system. Dave uses eight training heart rate zones (or intensities) in his training program.

The key is to find a training zone system that fits your needs and sport and to stick with a well-designed training program to increase your fitness and training performance.

Very Light or Daily-Activity Zone: 50 to 60 Percent of Maximal Heart Rate

This is the easiest intensity you can work out at and still improve your fitness. At this intensity your body is mostly using fat as a fuel for your working muscles. Most serious athletes feel guilty exercising at this intensity. Conversation is easy and there is no sensation of being out of breath. This is the long slow distance (LSD) training zone.

This pace is great for

1. beginning an exercise regime or starting out again after a layoff due to injury or illness,
2. recovery sessions, and
3. improving overall health.

Exercise for Health Zone: 60 to 70 Percent of Maximal Heart Rate

This could be called the "fitness zone" because this intensity level is excellent for strengthening your heart. This is the zone that works your heart hard enough for it to get stronger and ready for a steady, moderate pace.

This zone has many benefits:

1. It improves the ability of your heart to pump blood.
2. It increases the sum total of small blood vessels in your extremities.

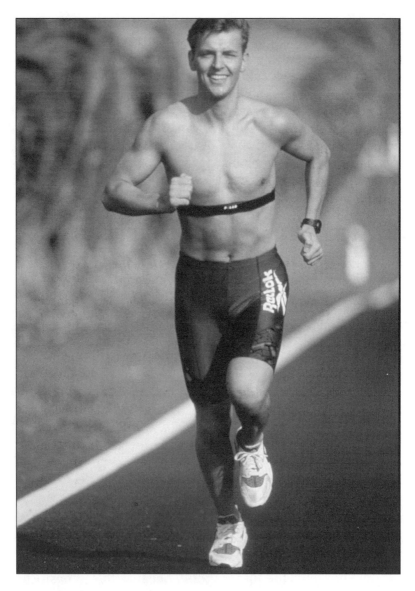

3. It increases the enzymes in your muscles that are responsible for oxygen metabolism.

4. It increases the cardiovascular capacity of your muscle tissues, tendons, and ligaments.

5. It improves your endurance.

6. It is right for people looking to expend energy at a moderate intensity.

Aerobic or Exercise for Fitness Training Zone: 70 to 85 Percent of Maximal Heart Rate

The aerobic zone is the standard training zone that for years has been referred to as "the target heart rate zone," since it is the most popular intensity for general fitness. This is often the fastest pace you can maintain and still remain comfortable and talk while exercising. It is called the steady state zone, as it is the fastest pace

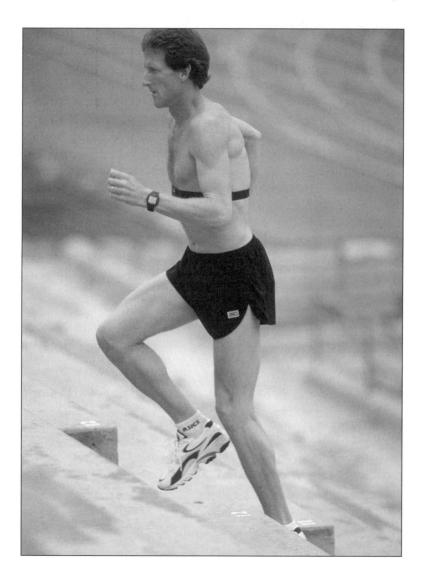

you can maintain for long periods of time (for most people). Lactic acid does not build up in this zone.

When you are unfit, your muscles will choose carbohydrate as their primary fuel, stored as glycogen in your muscles, during exercise at this intensity. As you become more fit, your body selects an increasing percentage of fat as its fuel, allowing you to race longer at this intensity while saving your limited stores of glycogen.

There are several benefits of training in this zone:

1. It improves endurance.
2. It "familiarizes" your body with a faster pace.
3. It begins to raise the speed you can maintain without building up lactate.

Improved-Performance Training Zone: 85 to 100 Percent of Maximal Heart Rate

At this level you are training near the point where aerobic training crosses over and becomes anaerobic training. At some point between 80 and 90 percent of your MHR, a very fit individual will be training at or near the anaerobic threshold. When you train within this range, the primary benefit is to increase your body's ability to metabolize lactic acid, allowing you to train harder before crossing over into the pain of lactate accumulation and oxygen debt.

If you were asked to describe the intensity of this level you would say that it is "hard." You are going to feel the pain that comes with training hard—tired muscles, heavy breathing, and fatigue. If you keep with it, though, in return the training effect will occur, and you will be able to sustain more work over longer amounts of time at lower heart rate levels.

The benefits of training at or near your anaerobic threshold are the following:

1. It increases your muscles' tolerance to lactic acid.
2. It increases the enzymes in your muscles that are responsible for anaerobic metabolism.
3. This is the pace used for racing, breakaways, time trialing, and running hills in a race.

At 90–100 percent of MHR, you have gone beyond your lactate (anaerobic) threshold and will be operating at a large oxygen deficit, meaning that your muscles will not be able to deliver the amount of oxygen they need to complete the work. Lactic acid will develop very quickly. Your body can tolerate efforts in this area of the zone only for short periods of time.

There are two major benefits of training in this area of the zone:

1. It increases your muscles' tolerance to very large amounts of lactic acid.

2. It helps improve your sprinting and hard, short-effort ability.

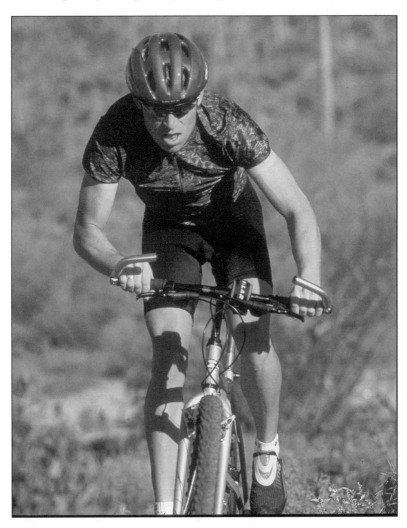

Why Training Lowers Heart Rate

Resting heart rate varies widely from athlete to athlete. A low heart rate is advantageous because it usually reflects a strong and highly efficient heart. A heart with a lower rate uses less energy than a heart with a faster rate if both pump the same amount of blood per minute.

Like heart rate, cardiac output (the amount of blood pumped per minute) at rest varies from person to person; but in general, a large person will have a greater resting cardiac output than a small person, and people of comparable size will have comparable cardiac outputs. In a trained person, resting heart rate declines as aerobic fitness increases; thus, the stroke volume must increase to maintain a consistent cardiac output.

A lower heart rate offers a physiological advantage. During an endurance event, a highly trained athlete's heart rate range (the difference between the lowest heart rate and the highest rate for any one person) is expanded. If your resting heart rate is low, your heart works more efficiently to pump more blood with each beat. Because of this, your heart may not have to reach as high a rate as that of someone who is less trained in order to perform a given activity. Or, it takes longer to reach the maximum exercise heart rate.

The underlying mechanisms that control the heart rate and stroke volume changes are not fully understood. The resting heart rate declines somewhat after only a few weeks of endurance training. The reduced heart rate allows a longer rest between beats, and more blood enters the ventricles (the chambers of the heart that pump the blood). This larger amount of blood stretches the heart muscle and leads to a stronger contraction and a greater ejection of blood. Eventually, as a result of prolonged endurance training, the heart becomes larger and stronger, and the heart rate decreases further.

At a given workload, the lower the heart rate, the higher the stroke volume, and the more aerobically fit the person.

Thus the resting heart rate can be used as a general indicator of aerobic illness. A better measure, however, is the heart rate at submaximal or maximal exercise. Training lowers the heart rate response during a standard amount of exercise. To get an accurate assessment of a person's fitness level, a standard submaximal or maximal exercise test must be carried out either in a laboratory or in the field under controlled conditions.

The Power of Heart Rate Training

Just as with the pros, a heart rate monitor can give you a physiological window into your body, through accurate heart rate measurement, and into your body's response to the moment-to-moment changes in physical effort.

"A heart rate monitor is an essential tool in your arsenal of exercise equipment," points out Skip Hamilton. "A heart rate monitor may be the most important accessory you could ever purchase for precision monitoring of training and competition intensities," he adds.

Now that you've seen the benefits of using a heart rate monitor in training and competition, in the next chapters you will learn more precisely how to use a heart rate monitor for a particular sport or activity. These chapters were written by some of the leading experts in the field. You need to experiment with their training suggestions. Learn their training principles and use your heart rate monitor to help revolutionize your training for health, fitness, and competition.

Finally, review all the chapters—and while you may consider yourself primarily a runner or a cyclist, there are probably some additional training tips and workout suggestions in the other chapters that can be applied to your favorite sport or activity.

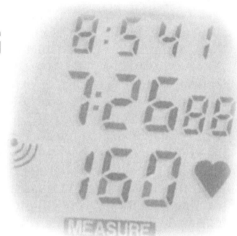

CHAPTER 3

WALKING

THERESE IKNOIAN

All you need to walk is a good pair of comfortable shoes, or so the saying goes. For the novice, that might be true. But as you get a little more serious about your walking program, a heart rate monitor becomes an essential part of your workout bag of tricks, since most walkers—no matter what level or how enthusiastic—don't have coaches or private trainers as other athletes, such as runners or cyclists, might have.

Using Your Heart Rate Monitor for Walking

Depending on your level and goal as a walker, your monitor will serve as your private trainer, exercise partner, coach, motivator, conscience, instructor, or even your personal nag, for example on days when you should do more, or less, than planned. Whatever role the monitor fills (and that role will change with the day or month), it will be an invaluable adjunct to getting where you want to be in your walking program.

Initially, you'll just need to get used to how your heart rate reacts to walking workouts of different types. What you'll notice, especially if you have experience in another sport or activity, is that your heart rate will likely be lower during walking at submaximal levels than at equivalent levels of perceived exertion and muscular force while running or cycling, for example. However, your maximal heart rate, if it has been tested in a laboratory and if you're an experienced walker, will likely be comparable to the rate you could elicit under laboratory test conditions at another activity.

As explained in chapter 1, heart rates vary with the activity, so take some time to experience yours at different speeds, on various terrains, or in different weather conditions.

Although your heart rate might be lower overall during some training conditions, you will probably find that seriously striding can be more intense than most people imagine. If you aren't used to monitoring your heart rate, whether manually or electronically, you'll probably be surprised how high it climbs even while you are not pushing yourself to near maximal effort. At least one study (Porcari, 1987, The Physician and Sportsmedicine) has shown that 9 of 10 women and at least two-thirds of men can reach a training heart rate, defined as equal to or greater than 70 percent of maximal, when asked to stride a mile briskly. Ten men in this study who had high levels of maximum oxygen consumption, and who had not reached training heart rates in the first mile, were then given a heart rate monitor and told to maintain a certain pulse rate. With a number to watch and push toward, these men were also able to achieve their training heart rates.

So to reach those percentages of your maximal heart rate for greater fitness and good health, or even higher for performance-training needs, you'll need to become muscularly efficient and technically sound as a walker. So take some time, as you're becoming acquainted with your heart rate monitor, to practice refined walking technique and economical use of your body to propel yourself forward. My book, *Walking Faster*, out in early 1998, has a thorough explanation with illustrations and photographs of the biomechanics of walking technique. As we'll briefly consider later, proper technique can be one way to adjust the intensity of your walking workouts.

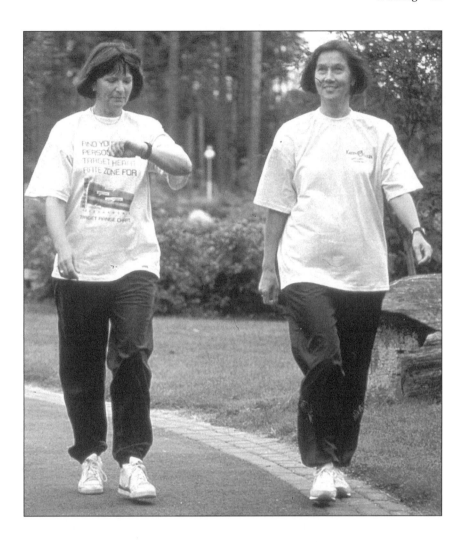

Finding Your Optimal Training Intensity for Walking

Before you can apply to your own training the physiologically based calculations of heart rate ranges, as explained in chapter 2, you'll need to establish your personal goals and your reasons for walking. It might be easy to mimic what a friend or spouse says his or her reason for regular walks is, but yours might be different or perhaps should be different. Unless you recognize your goals, setting up training intensities as part of a personalized walking program is like driving a car with your eyes closed. It's not effective, and you probably won't get where you want to go.

Know Your Goals

So let's take a look at possible reasons and goals for your walking program. Of course, you might find you have two or more reasons for walking, but try to determine which is your primary reason:

1. General health—Perhaps knowing you have a family history of a certain disease, for example high blood pressure or diabetes, or perhaps to stave off any potential risk of such a disease, you choose simply to walk regularly as an investment in your health. It's simpler than other activities and will accomplish the goal.

2. Weight loss—A large percentage of Americans are overweight or overfat, and they start walking either to lose weight or to keep weight off. Walking is low impact and is perfect as a nonstressful way to control your weight.

3. Aerobic fitness—Structuring appropriate walking workout intensities can build strong cardiovascular fitness, which will strengthen your heart, lungs, and entire vascular system.

4. Performance and competition—Whether you want to strongly walk local weekend events in your community or seriously race walk at some level from local to national, you can find the training intensity to help you along the way.

Primary goal: _____

Take a look at table 3.1. Find your primary goal on the far left and read across to the heart rate range and its corresponding rating of perceived exertion appropriate for your goal. Note that, especially if you are aiming for strong aerobic fitness or higher performance, you will not walk at this level every day, but every two to three days, depending on your program. Refer to the next section in this chapter for more details on program

TABLE 3.1	Zone Training: Comparison of Goals, Heart Rates, and RPE		
	Heart rate range (age based)	Rating of perceived exertion (Borg 6–20 scale)	Descriptive RPE
Zone 1 General health	50–60 percent	9–10	Very comfortable and light. Very conversational.
Zone 2 Weight control	60–70 percent	11–12	Fairly light. Brisk, but still comfortable. Breathing becomes slightly noticeable.
Zone 3 Aerobic fitness	70–80 percent	13–15	Somewhat hard, but ability to talk remains.
Zone 4 Performance	80–90 percent	16–17	Hard to very hard. Heavier breathing.
Zone 5 Competition	90–100 percent	18–20	Very hard to very fast. A real push. Quite heavy breathing.

design, and back to chapter 1 for more information on the intensity zones.

Know, too, that you will achieve some part of all four goals at all levels; for example, you will lose body weight and body fat doing workouts in higher zones, just as you'll achieve some amount of cardiovascular fitness in lower zones.

Evaluate Your Walking Fitness

Take one day to evaluate your current level of walking fitness by taking a one-mile walking test. Participating in this test assumes you have been active and have medical clearance for continuing activity.

One-Mile Walking Test

This test involves walking one measured mile, preferably on a school track in the inside lane because of distance accuracy, as fast as you can. (If the track is 400 meters, rather than 440 yards, you'll walk about 9 meters farther than four laps to complete one mile.) Wearing your heart rate monitor, warm up thoroughly for at least five minutes and stretch. Include a few short walking sprints just before you're ready to start. Know what 90 percent of your maximal heart rate is, because our goal here is not to test your maximum oxygen consumption but to do an informal evaluation of your speed by allowing you to go as fast as you can while continuing to work primarily aerobically. Therefore, if your heart rate begins to climb over 90 percent, pull back slightly.

Toe the starting line in the first lane. Hit "start" on a stopwatch, or on your heart rate monitor if it has that function, as you cross the line on your first step. Try to pace yourself, walking hard throughout, but not starting so fast that you can't hold on to the pace. You shouldn't start so fast that you die off at the end; you should in fact have a little oomph left to try to sprint at the finish. Maintain good technique. Either record your heart rate every lap (or more frequently if your monitor can do that) or take a quick look and remember the numbers.

When you finish one mile, hit "stop" on your stopwatch, and continue to watch your monitor for a few seconds while you keep moving to get a final reading of your highest heart rate. Keep walking to allow yourself to cool down.

Note your time for future comparisons.

One-mile time: _____

Note your heart rate (HR) progression, its percentage of your age-graded maximum (percentage of MHR) and related rating of perceived exertion (RPE), and also, for future reference, the highest HR achieved.

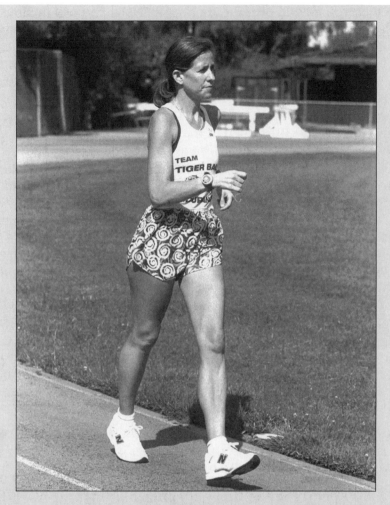

First-lap HR/percentage of MHR/RPE: _____/_____ /_____

Second-lap HR/percentage of MHR/RPE: _____/_____/_____

Third-lap HR/percentage of MHR/RPE: _____/_____ /_____

Fourth-lap (final) HR/percentage of MHR/RPE: _____/_____/_____

Highest HR seen/percentage of MHR: _____/_____

Retake the one-mile evaluation every four to eight weeks so you have a good idea of how you are progressing. Likely, your speed will increase while your HR and RPE remain the same.

Once you've completed the one-mile walk, you will be able to more closely pinpoint your current—note that important word—optimal training intensity by cross-checking your goal with your one-mile evaluation of your walking fitness. Look again to table 3.1 for an illustration of training intensities.

For example, if your goal is higher aerobic fitness or walking performance, but your walking fitness level as demonstrated by your heart rates and perceived exertion in the one-mile test places you below those heart rate ranges, you'll need to spend some time walking in the lower zones to build fitness so you can advance toward your goal. But if your walking fitness level is within the higher zones, you're ready to tackle a structured program, using those ranges as your guide.

Now you can more clearly see how your monitor becomes a coach, private trainer, and educator.

One more word: Unless your maximal heart rate and maximum oxygen consumption have been laboratory tested, these heart rates calculated are only estimates and may be significantly higher or lower. As you begin using a monitor on your walks, note your level of perceived exertion to see if it matches that of the range. If not, you might find your personal maximal heart rate to be higher or lower, and you'll need to adjust your workout heart rates up or down.

Designing Your Walking Program

Now you know the zone within which you are able to perform your walking workouts. If that corresponds to your goal, all the better. If it's lower than your goal, your monitor will let you know when you're ready to move on. For example, you will notice your walks getting longer or faster while your heart rate stays the same or even drops. If you retake the one-mile evaluation, you'll notice you were faster with the same heart rate—or perhaps you didn't go faster, but your heart rate was lower. Keep thorough records so you can analyze your progression over time.

Walks in the Workout Zones

Refer to table 3.2 for an overview of walking workouts that are suitable and recommended for each zone's fitness levels and goals. Obviously, all walks in all zones will encourage weight loss and improvements in cardiovascular fitness and health, and will help you walk faster and stronger. For specific goals, it would be best to concentrate your workouts in that zone.

TABLE 3.2	Walking Workout Samples by Zone		
	Duration	**Frequency**	**Comments**
Zone 1	20–30 minutes, minimum	3–5 days a week, minimum	Could take shorter walks but walk twice per day, if desired.
Zone 2	45–60 minutes	At least 5 days a week	Consider walking daily for optimal weight loss and/or control.
Zone 3	20–60 minutes	3–5 days a week	Combine with workouts from zones 1–2 for 5–7 walks per week.
Zone 4	15–45 total minutes per workout	1–2 days a week, maximum	(1) Combine with workouts from zones 1–3 for 6–7 walks per week. (2) Shorter walks are at a higher HR percentage, and vice versa. May break into 2–3 intervals with short rests.
Zone 5	15–25 total minutes per workout	1–2 days a week, maximum	(1) Same as above. (2) Workouts are combinations of intervals of 1–5 minutes, with rest between each of 1–5 minutes.

Zone 1

Since your goal is primarily to achieve solid overall health benefits, walk at least 20–30 minutes three to five days a week. If you walk shorter distances, then walk more frequently; if you walk longer distances, you may walk less frequently. If you find that even 20–30 minutes is difficult, you can occasionally walk an even shorter time, say 10 minutes, but do that two to three times a day to reach the recommended total.

Monitor application: Use the monitor to push you slightly so you can achieve your heart rates quickly on your shorter walks.

Zone 2

With weight control as the primary goal, you will want to walk a minimum of five days a week and up to seven days a week. Keep your pace steady and purposeful, using your arms and legs strongly. At a brisk four mile per hour pace (15-minute miles), a 140-pound person can use about 235 calories in 45 minutes.

Monitor application: Use the monitor to make sure you don't walk so fast that you are unable to sustain the length of your walk to achieve and maintain optimal weight goals.

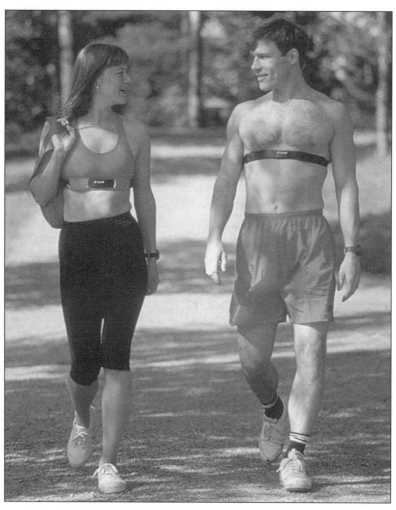

Should You Speed Up to Slim Down?

Edmund R. Burke

Myth: Performing aerobic exercise at low intensity promotes a greater loss of body fat than exercising at high intensity does. For years it has been the prevailing notion that slower is better when it comes to weight loss, or "fat burning."

Fact: Can you imagine being told that you can ride, run, or swim faster to lose weight? On the surface, that statement might seem to resemble one of those ad gimmicks that promises you an elimination of body fat while you sleep, or some similarly wild, unrealistic claim. However, if you truly understand the intricate manner in which your metabolism operates, the previous statement does not appear nearly as outrageous.

For years, we in the exercise science community have been telling you to exercise at less than 60% of $\dot{V}O_2$max to burn fat (70% of MHR). Exercising at higher intensities, we told you, forces your muscles to burn glycogen (stored carbohydrate), leaving your fat stores intact. Although the concept of keeping exercise intensity low in order to mobilize and selectively burn a higher percentage of fat may sound logical, it does not add up mathematically, and, more important, has never been verified in the laboratory.

When you exercise at 50% of your $\dot{V}O_2$max (65% of your MHR), your body fat stores will provide about 50% of your energy needs. On the other hand, when you raise your intensity to 75% of max $\dot{V}O_2$ (85% of MHR), fat will provide 33% of the calories needed to pedal, run, or swim. With these numbers, it sounds like slower exercising will be better for weight loss.

Let the truth be known: You can burn more calories by exercising faster—and better yet, burn just as much fat—by exercising at a higher heart rate intensity. I'll show you why.

→

Slower exercising only appears superior if you neglect to look at the total amount of calories burned during your workout. Data collected in the laboratory should help to illustrate this point. In a study conducted at the University of Texas, Dr. Jack Wilmore and Dave Costill found that moderately fit cyclists exercising at 50% of their $\dot{V}O_2$max burned approximately 220 calories during 30 minutes of exercising. But when they raised the intensity to 75% of $\dot{V}O_2$max, the cyclists' caloric cost went up to about 330 calories (these results were reported in their book *Physiology of Sport and Exercise*). Without using your calculator, you can see that 50% of 220 and 33% of 330 calories will give you 110 calories burned. In other words, 30 minutes of exercising burns the same amount of fat! However, at 75% of $\dot{V}O_2$max, you burn over 100 more calories in the 30 minutes of exercise. So, if your goal is to get leaner, your bottom line should be total calorie burning.

Owen Anderson, PhD, reports in *Running Research News* that if you have only 30 minutes to work out and you want to lose weight and increase your fitness, you are better off working out at 75–80% of max $\dot{V}O_2$ (83–88% of MHR), an intensity level that a fit individual should be able to maintain for 30 minutes. In fairness, he points out that if you work out at a lower intensity of 50% of max $\dot{V}O_2$ for just 15 minutes longer, you will consume as many calories as in the faster workout. However, since this is a slow pace, if the 75% max $\dot{V}O_2$ pace could be carried on for an extra 15 minutes, you would burn about 50% more calories. For workouts of routine duration, lower-intensity exercising does not break down more fat, and you will expend far fewer calories than if you were to ride, swim, or run at a higher intensity.

If your goals are to improve your cardiovascular system and to lose weight, your aim should be to maximize your total energy expenditure. The preceding example shows that this is best accomplished via higher-intensity exercising. A realistic level of exertion would be 70–80% of $\dot{V}O_2$max (80–88% of maximal heart rate), an intensity you are more likely to maintain for 30 minutes.

There is another reason to cruise along at a higher intensity while riding, running, or swimming to ensure fat loss, according to Jackie Berning, RD, sports nutritionist at the University of Colorado at Colorado Springs: "After exercise, when you eat your next meal, you begin to replenish both carbohydrates and fat in your muscles. As soon as excess calories (from either carbohydrates or fat) exit, your body will begin to store them as fat. If you exercise at an intensity that burns more fat than carbohydrates, you will rapidly replenish your carbohydrate stores. The net result is that the caloric excess of carbohydrates will have to be stored as fat. Thus, it means that you have not altered your body's overall energy balance."

Keep in mind that you lose weight and body fat when you burn more calories through exercising than you have consumed, not because you burn fat or carbohydrate or protein when you exercise.

Does low-intensity exercise have *any* role in weight loss? Of course it does. But you must look at the goal of your exercise program. If your goal is just to improve your overall health, exercising at any intensity is beneficial. The recent recommendation published jointly by the American College of Sports Medicine and the Centers for Disease Control, which supports the concept of moderate exercise, is that all of us need to get at least 30 minutes of moderate-intensity activity most days of the week.

Remember, low-intensity exercise does have one advantage: you can exercise for longer periods of time. Whereas you may be able to exercise only for short periods of time at 75% of $\dot{V}O_2$max or above, most of us can ride, run, or swim for hours at 50–60% of $\dot{V}O_2$max , and the total number of calories and fat calories used would be greater. But for many people time is at a premium; so, there's no reason to slow down unless you are training for a long race or need an easy workout.

If your goal is to get leaner, the bottom line is to cycle, swim, or run at the highest intensity that you can maintain for 30 minutes or longer. You need not give consideration to the type of fuel burned during an activity to guide your exercise prescription. Until proven otherwise, when it comes to weight loss, a calorie burned is a calorie burned, regardless of its origin.

Zone 3

This zone builds aerobic fitness when your heart rate is kept within the range recommended, taking walks three to five days a week. If you want to work out more than that, walk alternating days at a lower intensity. For lifelong fitness, one could choose walks almost exclusively from this zone and remain fit and healthy.

Monitor application: Use the monitor to keep you steady, as well as to keep you in zone 3 on your hard days and to keep you at lower levels on the other days.

Zone 4

Nearly the highest level for attaining performance, this range is strictly for veteran walkers who want to build speed and enhance athletic ability, with an eye to possible competition at some level. Walks at this high level are done only one to two times a week, with less experienced walkers limiting themselves to once a week. They should never be done on back-to-back days, but instead should always be followed by two to three days of walks with heart rates kept in lower zones.

Monitor application: Use the monitor as a hard-driving coach to push you strongly on your zone 4 days but to keep you honestly at easy levels on your recovery days.

Zone 5

Used only by veteran walkers seeking peak performance and competition, workouts in this area are kept to short intervals with plenty of rest between each one. As in zone 4, walking workouts in this zone are limited for safety to one to two days a week and are never done back-to-back with another workout from zone 4 or 5. Follow with two to three days of easy workouts from the lower zones or even a day off.

Monitor application: Of particular interest will be how quickly your heart rate drops during recoveries between intervals. The more quickly it drops, the higher your fitness level.

Note that those able to walk in zones 3, 4, and 5 might want to incorporate one long walk into their program each week. Each long walk should cover up to a third of the week's total mileage, for example, 7–8 miles if you normally cover about 25 miles a week. Because their length is what makes them more difficult, long walks will be done at about 65–75 percent of your maximal heart rate. See page 57 for a Sample Training Week for the Moderate Walker.

TRAINING PLAN

SAMPLE TRAINING WEEK FOR THE MODERATE WALKER

MONDAY

Steady walk, 2 1/2 miles, in zone 2 (60–70 percent of MHR, RPE 11–12).

TUESDAY

Rest.

WEDNESDAY

Four-mile steady walk in zone 3 (70–80 percent of MHR, RPE 13–15).

THURSDAY

Rest.

FRIDAY

Three-mile steady walk with speed play.

Do one-minute comfortably fast bursts (zone 4, 80–90 percent of MHR, RPE 16–17) with two minutes of steady walking (zone 3, 70–80 percent of MHR, RPE 13–15) between each burst, four to six bursts per walk.

SATURDAY

Rest.

SUNDAY

Five-mile steady walk in zone 2 (60–70 percent of MHR, RPE 11–12).

Total: 14 1/2 miles

Note: Adapted from "Fitness Walking".

Warm-Ups and Cool-Downs

Don't forget to use your heart rate monitor as a tool to help you warm up and cool down properly before and after each walk.

During your warm-ups, watch the numbers to keep them starting low; then pick up your pace gradually over the first three to eight minutes of your walk until you reach the appropriate training zone. If you are doing a zone 4 walk, spend a little longer in your warm-up, finishing it with some fast sprints that push you to 80 percent or beyond.

For cool-down, gradually slow down your walking pace until your heart rate reaches about 60 percent or less. After your walk, stretch well. For a guide to recommended stretches for walkers, see *Walking Fast* (1998) or *Fitness Walking* (1995).

Cross-Training

No matter how dedicated, walkers cannot live by walks alone. And if you're traveling, injured, or inhibited by weather, you might be forced to find alternatives to your walks.

If you've scheduled an easy or off day, you may participate in another activity, but make sure of two things: that it won't make you too sore to walk well the next day, and that you continue to observe your heart rate and keep it low. Your body doesn't know if it's walking, only at what level it's working, so if the day is supposed to be an easy one, keep it easy.

Same goes for hard workout days: If you choose to do something other than walk—perhaps because you're on vacation or the weather forces you into a health club—keep your heart rate in your chosen range and you'll get nearly the same cardiovascular workout, although the muscles you work might be different if the activity stresses you differently biomechanically.

You then could choose cross-training activities with two purposes. Either you want a totally different muscular workout to give your walking muscles a break, for example on an off day, or you want a muscular workout more similar to walking, for example on a scheduled walking day when you can't get to it. For workouts that use muscles mostly in different ways, choose cycling (indoors or out), weight lifting, stretching, hilly hiking, downhill skiing, swimming, or group exercise such as aerobics or step classes. For workouts that use muscles in mostly similar ways, choose running, stationary stair climbing, mostly flat hiking, cross-country skiing (indoors or out), deep-water running, shallow-water walking, or treadmill walking.

Remember, like many cardiovascular workouts, walking doesn't significantly improve upper-body strength or overall flexibility. Therefore, walkers should choose a variety of resistance workouts two to three times a week to strengthen their muscles in order to increase walking strength as well as to lessen the chance of injury or strain. Walkers should also stretch before and after every walk, as well as on their off days, if possible.

Adjusting Intensity in Your Walking Workouts

Walkers don't have to rely only on slowing down or speeding up to decrease or increase the intensity of a workout. In fact, until walkers are extremely proficient at proper technique, some might find it difficult to push their heart rates to 75–90 percent of their maximum while relying only on speed.

Let's take a look at several methods to vary the intensity of your walk, concluding, of course, with a few pointers on technique.

Terrain

Flat trails and roads of concrete and asphalt aren't the only places to walk.

Walking up inclines, hills, or stairs can increase your energy expenditure by 50 percent or more because of the additional muscular contractions needed to push you upward against gravity's constant pull downward. Avoid leaning forward from the waist, keep your abdominals tight, and use your buttocks and calves to push strongly as you move upward. Also use your arms, bent at a 90-degree angle at the elbow, to help power you up the hill. Novice walkers should avoid hills, or should take plenty of breaks as they climb, to keep the heart rate from shooting up too high.

If you walk on a treadmill, you can use hills to your advantage, perhaps alternating short inclines with zero grade to control your walk's intensity. Any surface that is soft will also increase the intensity of your walk without mandating more speed. The softer the surface and the more you have to use increased muscle to power yourself forward, the more energy you will expend. For example, grassy surfaces, such as a stadium infield, can increase intensity by a third, while sand and soft dirt can double your energy use and soft snow can triple it.

Environment

Walking against wind can also increase your calorie expenditure. Interestingly, studies show that if you are forced to work twice as hard while fighting the wind in one direction on a track, you won't cut that workload in half as you walk with the wind at your back.

Shoes

Some competition walkers have been known to wear training shoes that are slightly heavier and then switch in races to light-weight shoes. Because turnover—the number of steps you take per minute—is faster in walking than in running, requiring more muscular contractions per minute, a couple of ounces added to or taken off your feet can increase or decrease your walk's intensity slightly.

Duration

If time is on your side, walk farther and longer, even if only once a week. A strong walker could tackle a two- or three-hour walk or hike on weekends, since the length will force the body to use more fat as an energy source.

Speed

Even if you don't have the technique to go faster for your entire walk, you could incorporate short sprints every few minutes (called "fartlek" or speed play). Start with sprints that are no longer than you can accomplish with good technique (even if only 15 or 20 seconds); walk easy enough for a long enough time between sprints to allow your heart rate to return to its normal pace during your walk, and then do it again. As you become stronger and more efficient, your sprints will get longer or faster.

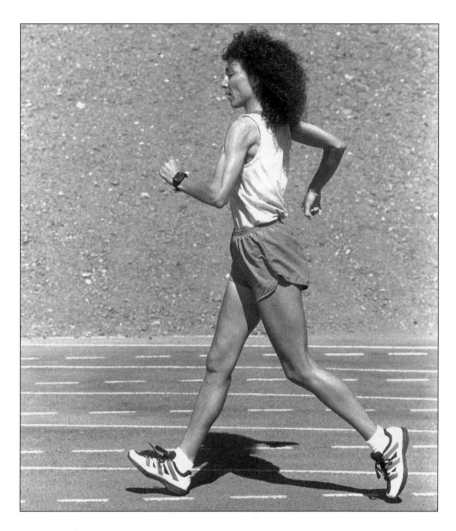

Technique

A full discussion of technique here is impossible, but take note of these three pointers. Incorporating these tips will help you use speed to increase the intensity of your walk and help you avoid injury at any pace:

- **Feet.** Try to move your feet faster, taking more steps per minute rather than taking long ground-swallowing strides. Be light on your feet.

- **Arms.** Bend your arms 90 degrees at the elbow and pump them strongly, using your back muscles to power you forward. Keep your shoulders relaxed and elbows tucked in to your waist.

- **Push-off.** Use a strong contraction of the muscles up the back of your leg and buttocks to push your toes firmly against the ground to propel you forward. Feel your leg extend behind you from the hip and sense the ground under your toes.

What about carrying hand weights to increase intensity? Studies have shown that you can do yourself more good, and put yourself at less chance of injury, by speeding up your tempo as opposed to clutching weights. Unless you swing the hand weights quite vigorously to shoulder height or even higher, the number of extra calories used can be small. Yet you've not only fatigued your upper body with the result that you might need to cut short your walk, you've probably also thrown off your personal stride, perhaps strained a muscle, and in addition may be raising your blood pressure because you have to grip the weights.

If you want to up the intensity, forget weights, and just choose either more speed or one of the other six techniques already discussed.

Taking Walking to the Next Level

The beauty of walking is its simplicity: All you have to do is step out the front door—and anyone of any fitness level can find success. Just as with many activities, however, you can also step up its level athletically or competitively.

Whether power walking in your community's local marathon or racewalking with an eye on legal technique, you will find opportunities to move up a notch or two as your training dictates. With a monitor "coaching" you, you'll have a better idea of what you are capable of and when you should try it.

If you're interested in the next level, select an appropriate goal—the weekend 5K (3.1 miles) fun run in three months or a judged race walk next year—and then train accordingly. You'll likely need to become more structured in your workouts, following physiologic training guidelines and using your monitor to keep you on target. *Walking Fast* also lays out distinct programs for various walking levels and goals, applying heart rate as one way to measure intensity to achieve success.

TRAINING PLAN

SAMPLE TRAINING WEEK
FOR THE PERFORMANCE WALKER

MONDAY

Rest.

TUESDAY

Five-mile walk.

Warm up for one mile, progressing from zone 1 to 3.

For the workout, walk three miles. Complete three intervals of one mile each (zone 4, 80–90 percent of MHR, RPE 16–17) with three to four minutes' rest, allowing your MHR to drop to 65–70 percent with an RPE of 11–12 between each interval.

Cool down with one-mile walk in zone 2.

WEDNESDAY

Four-mile steady walk in zone 2 (60–70 percent of MHR, RPE 11–12).

THURSDAY

Three-mile steady walk in zone 3 (70–80 percent of MHR, RPE 13–15).

FRIDAY

Four-mile steady walk with speed play.

Do eight 90-second bursts of very fast walking (zone 5, 90–100 percent of MHR, RPE 18–20) with 90 seconds' rest between each burst (zone 3, 70–80 percent of MHR, RPE 13–15).

SATURDAY

Rest

SUNDAY

Seven-mile steady walk in zone 2 (60–70 percent of MHR, RPE 11–12).

Total: 23 miles

Note: Adapted from *Walking Fast*.

Briefly, a walker will need to add a long walk for increased endurance every 7–10 days at 65–75 percent of maximal, one to two walks each week designed to increase lactate threshold (either 30–45 minutes continuous or 5–20-minute intervals at approximately 80–85 percent), and, to increase oxygen consumption and biomechanical efficiency, shorter intervals of 2–5 minutes at 90–100 percent with very easy walking between each. See page 63 for a Sample Training Week for the Performance Walker. To reach the next level, refined technique, as briefly addressed earlier, will be a top priority.

Walking Resources

If you are interested in racewalking, contact the national office of USA Track & Field (PO Box 120, Indianapolis, IN 46206; 317-261-0478) to learn the telephone number of your area's association office. Your area office can direct you to the local racewalking chairperson who will know about events, races, classes, and instruction. USA Track & Field is the national governing body of track, field, long-distance running, and racewalking.

Another resource is *Walking* magazine, a national consumer magazine that addresses not only general health and weight-loss concerns, but also technique and training for all levels and walking news. The magazine also runs a calendar of selected national events.

Learning to correctly and effectively monitor and track your heart rate will not only make walking more enjoyable but also allow you to reach your goals. Every walk becomes a challenge with a personal trainer strapped to your wrist.

CHAPTER 4

RUNNING

ROY BENSON

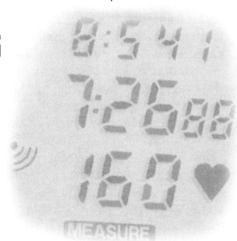

At first, track coaches thought it was just a matter of becoming better scientists as the discipline of exercise physiology came out of the lab and onto the athletic fields. The linear logic behind monitoring increasing levels of exercise intensity by counting pulse rates had a lot of appeal. At least it did to me, a younger distance-running coach without the years of experience needed to be good at practicing the "art" of coaching distance runners. Well, if I couldn't be much of an artist, at least I could quickly become a struggling scientist. Hence, I left high school teaching and coaching for grad school at the University of Florida to pursue a master's degree in PE, with emphasis in Exercise Physiology. As a grad assistant track coach in charge of the half-milers, I soon became a proponent of effort-based training (EBT), the concept of measuring workload intensity as well as pace.

Unfortunately, it was not easy to implement EBT principles because the telemetric heart rate monitor (HRM) had not yet escaped the confines of the cardiac rehab laboratories. To use EBT, about all I could do was count carotid artery pulses to measure how hard or easy my runners were practicing. The only equipment available was my low-rent index finger and my trusty old stopwatch. Furthermore, opportunities to count heart rates were pretty much limited to interval workouts at the track.

Finally, in the mid-1980s, our prayers were answered. Telemetric HRMs from Finland suddenly appeared, displaying beats per minute with great accuracy, although the product dependability of those early models left much to be desired. But after several years of constant refinement and improvements, current models are like the Energizer bunny: they just keep on going and going for years before they wear down.

However, since the very beginning of monitored training, a different problem has hampered the effective usage of HRMs. The availability of software (the info needed to make effective use of these electronic marvels) has not matched the availability and attractiveness of the hardware. So, in 1994 I leaped into the vacuum. I wrote my book *The Runner's Coach* and my booklet *Precision Running* (available from Polar) to help coaches, runners, and joggers understand the principles of EBT and know just what to do with their HRMs once they had them out of the package.

Now it's time for an update. We have discovered that we can't rely exclusively on the linear logic of exercise physiology to trust that the readings on our HRMs are always 100 percent meaningful. We've discovered that we can't be slaves to our monitors without risk of under- or overtraining—just like runners who rely only on their stopwatches for feedback. We have realized that intelligent use of our monitors also requires some understanding of exercise cardiology.

So, from an old coach, working in the trenches trying every day to correlate beats per minute with minutes per mile, here are my latest conclusions. Hang in there with me as I try to connect everything together with some old-fashioned common sense known as Coachly Wisdom.

Finding Your Optimal Training Intensity for Running

One of the first things I discovered was that runners really need to train at percentages of their maximal oxygen consumption, not simply at percentages of their maximal heart rate (MHR). It's too complicated to go into here, but trust that the Target Heart Rate (THR) Calculator (fig. 4.1, a and b) is designed to make that conversion for you. (For your convenience, however, I will still

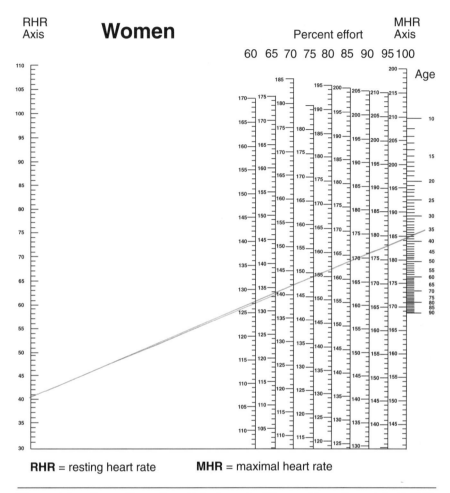

RHR Axis

Women

Percent effort

MHR Axis

60 65 70 75 80 85 90 95 100

Age

RHR = resting heart rate   **MHR** = maximal heart rate

Figure 4.1a Target Heart Rate Calculator for Women. Note: Copyright © 1991, 1993 by Roy Benson.

refer to your THR zones as percentages of MHR.) To use it, you need to know only two things: your morning resting heart rate (RHR) and your actual, or at least predicted, MHR.

At this point, permit me another short aside to explain why the numbers the calculator produces may be significantly different from what you are used to seeing. Different studies published in the last few years by Hakki, Pollack, Leger, Blair, and Kaminsky et al. have suggested that the venerable formula of 220 minus your age is no longer the best way to predict MHRs, especially for "chronically" fit adults. Therefore, my Target HR Calculator incorporates the work of all the above scientists by combining a logarithmic formula

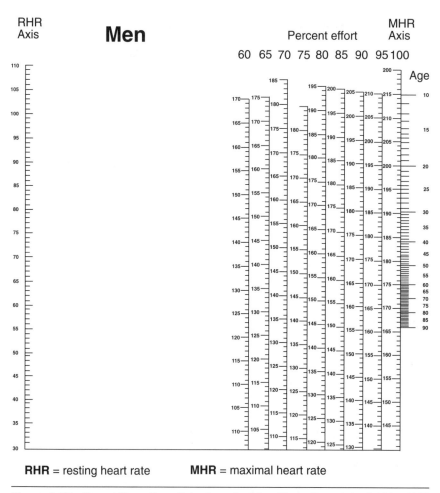

Figure 4.1b Target Heart Rate Calculator for Men. Note: Copyright © 1991, 1993 by Roy Benson.

devised by my colleague Larry Simpson to expand on the original work by Ned Frederick, PhD. Ned developed the original nomogram that so brilliantly featured the Karvonen formula, which gives credit for one's current level of fitness by incorporating resting heart rate.

See chapter 1 for suggestions to determine your RHR. Then locate and mark that number on the outside of the left-hand axis on the THR Calculator. Before deciding on a number for your MHR, bear in mind this startling fact: as much as 10 percent of the population could be as many as 24 beats per minute over or under their predicted MHR. Once you digest that little surprise, it's extremely important to understand something else: *your MHR doesn't*

*have anything to do with how good looking, smart, or rich you are, what
level of shape you're in, or how fast you are!* People's hearts have
different sizes. Smaller ones are wired to beat more frequently. Larger
ones beat more slowly because they eject more blood with each
stroke. That's important to understand so you will not feel bad if you
ever make the mistake of comparing your MHR to someone else's. Like
salaries, MHRs—and also THRs—should not be mentioned in polite
company. For the most part, your MHR can be accurately predicted by
simply matching it with age as I have done with the Calculator. Just find
your number of years on the outside edge of the right-hand axis.
Across from it, on the inside edge of this axis, is your predicted MHR.
Even though you can estimate your MHR, for a more accurate measure
I strongly recommend that you perform one of the stress tests
presented later in the chapter to determine your true MHR.

If you're not content to gamble that your heart is of average size,
I have some suggestions for determining whether your MHR is a
standard deviation or two above or below average.

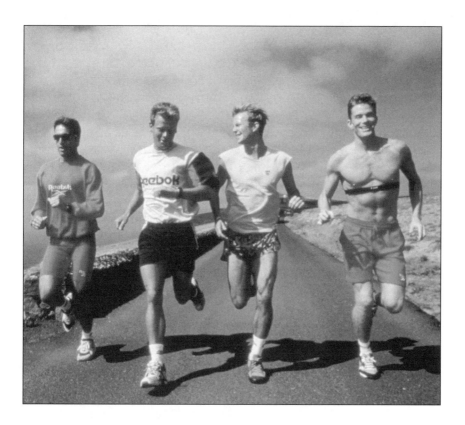

Coach Benson's Low-Rent, Low-Risk, Minimal Stress Test

If okay with your doctor, take this simple field test by going to a running track and timing yourself for one mile while jogging very slowly at the THRs you find for yourself from the 60–65 percent columns on my THR Calculator. Once you've finished that exciting task, jog another mile at 70–75 percent effort. Then use my Pace and Effort Chart (table 4.1) to see if there is a commonsense correlation between your current level of fitness and your THRs. Find your test times in the fourth and fifth columns from the left. They're the columns that show values for maintenance and recovery at 60–65 percent effort and values for phase I endurance pace at 70–75 percent. Ideally, your times for these two different mile trials should be on the same horizontal line. Then look across the line underneath your times to the columns on the left to see if there is any chance that your performance predicts what kind of shape you're in for 10K, 5K, or one mile. Is there a reasonable match? If your paces were way too slow or far too fast, perhaps your MHR is as much as one or two standard deviations above or below average. If you ran too hard and fast, lower your predicted MHR on the THR Calculator by as much as 24 beats per minute. Conversely, raise it by up to 24 beats per minute if your pace was so slow that you almost had to walk to keep from exceeding your 65 percent upper target limit. Try the test again to see if your times match up better. If all of this makes no sense, go ahead and pay a running cardiologist or a research physiologist to get a full, maximal exercise stress test on a treadmill. Or, with your cardiologist's permission, try this other field test. Keep in mind that both the first test I described and the next one are not validated by scientific research. I'm just using some coachly logic here.

TABLE 4.1 Coach Roy Benson's Four-Phase Training Pace and Effort Chart

If your current mile time is	Or if your current 5K time is	Or if your current 10K time is	And your maintenance and recovery pace will result in a 60–65% effort for each mile	And your phase I endurance pace will result in a 70–75% effort for each mile	And your phase II stamina pace will result in an 80–85% effort for each mile	And your phase III economy pace will result in a 90–95% effort for each 400 meters	And your phase IV speed pace will result in a 95–100% effort for each 100 meters
03:45	13:00 (04:11/mi)	27:00 (04:21/mi)	05:51	05:30	04:42	01:01.9	00:13.0
03:54	13:29 (04:21/mi)	28:00 (04:30/mi)	06:03	05:42	04:52	01:04.1	00:13.4
04:02	13:58 (04:30/mi)	29:00 (04:41/mi)	06:15	05:53	05:02	01:06.2	00:13.8
04:11	14:27 (04:39/mi)	30:00 (04:50/mi)	06:27	06:05	05:11	01:08.3	00:14.2
04:20	14:56 (04:49/mi)	31:00 (05:00/mi)	06:40	06:16	05:21	01:10.5	00:14.6
04:28	15:25 (04:58/mi)	32:00 (05:10/mi)	06:52	06:28	05:31	01:12.6	00:15.1
04:37	15:54 (05:07/mi)	33:00 (05:19/mi)	07:04	06:39	05:41	01:14.8	00:15.6
04:46	16:23 (05:18/mi)	34:00 (05:29/mi)	07:16	06:51	05:51	01:16.9	00:16.0
04:54	16:52 (05:26/mi)	35:00 (05:39/mi)	07:28	07:02	06:00	01:19.1	00:16.5
05:03	17:21 (05:35/mi)	36:00 (05:49/mi)	07:40	07:14	06:10	01:21.2	00:16.9
05:12	17:49 (05:45/mi)	37:00 (05:58/mi)	07:52	07:25	06:20	01:23.3	00:17.4
05:21	18:18 (05:54/mi)	38:00 (06:08/mi)	08:04	07:36	06:30	01:25.5	00:17.8
05:29	18:47 (06:03/mi)	39:00 (06:17/mi)	08:16	07:48	06:39	01:27.6	00:18.3

TABLE 4.1 (continued)

05:38	19:16 (06:13/mi)	40.00 (06:27/mi)	08:28	07:59	06:49	01:29.7	00:18.7
05:47	19:45 (06:22/mi)	41.00 (06:37/mi)	08:40	08:10	06:59	01:31.8	00:19.1
05:56	20:14 (06:31/mi)	42.00 (06:46/mi)	08:52	08:21	07:09	01:33.9	00:19.6
06:04	20:43 (06:41/mi)	43:00 (06:56/mi)	09:03	08:32	07:18	01:36.1	00:20.0
06:13	21:11 (06:50/mi)	44:00 (07:06/mi)	09:15	08:43	07:28	01:38.2	00:20.5
06:22	21:41 (06:59/mi)	45:00 (07:16/mi)	09:27	08:54	07:37	01:40.3	00:20.9
06:31	22:10 (07:09/mi)	46:00 (07:25/mi)	09:38	09:05	07:47	01:42.5	00:21.4
06:39	22:38 (07.18/mi)	47:00 (07:35/mi)	09:50	09:16	07:56	01:44.6	00:21.8
06:48	23:07 (07:27/mi)	48:00 (07:44/mi)	10:01	09:27	08:06	01:46.7	00:22.2
06:57	23:36 (07:37/mi)	49:00 (07:54/mi)	10:13	09:38	08:15	01:48.8	00:22.6
07:06	24:05 (07:46/mi)	50:00 (08:04/mi)	10:24	09:49	08:25	01:50.9	00:23.1
07:15	24:34 (07:55/mi)	51:00 (08:14/mi)	10:35	10:00	08:34	01:52.9	00:23.5
07:23	25:03 (08:05/mi)	52:00 (08:23/mi)	10:46	10:10	08:44	01:55.0	00:24.0
07:32	25:32 (08:14/mi)	53:00 (08:33/mi)	10:58	10:21	08:53	01:57.1	00:24.4
07:41	26:01 (08:24/mi)	54:00 (08:43/mi)	11:09	10:32	09:02	01:59.1	00:24.8
07:50	26:30 (08:33/mi)	55:00 (08:52/mi)	11:20	10:42	09:12	02:02.4	00:25.5
07:59	26:59 (08:42/mi)	56:00 (09:02/mi)	11:31	10:53	09:21	02:03.3	00:25.7
08:07	27:28 (08:51/mi)	57:00 (09:11/mi)	11:42	11:03	09:30	02:05.3	00:26.1
08:16	27:56 (09:01/mi)	58:00 (09:21/mi)	11:52	11:13	09:39	02:07.4	00:26.5
08:25	28:25 (09:10/mi)	59:00 (09:31/mi)	12:03	11:24	09:48	02:09.4	00:27.0
08:34	28:54 (09:19/mi)	60:00 (09:41/mi)	12:14	11:34	09:57	02:11.4	00:27.4

Compiled by: Larry Simpson. References: Separately published research of J. Daniels & M.J. Karvonen; also "The Perfect Pace," Runner's World (Amby Burfoot).

Coach Benson's Low-Rent, High-Risk, Maximal Stress Test

This field test, again with permission of your doctor, requires some racing experience so you can make an honest estimate of how fast you can currently run a two-mile time trial on the track. Relax, you don't have to actually run an all-out two-mile time trial. You just need to know how fast you would be likely to average per each 400-meter lap. So, take a guess: how fast could you run eight laps around a track? Good. Now divide that total time into 400-meter splits. Then, duplicate the protocol of a couple of well-known treadmill maximal stress tests by doing the following test while checking your heart monitor at the end of each of the first six laps and then every 100 meters of the last two laps. You will need to carry a separate stopwatch in each hand so you can simply time each lap and not have to worry about doing the math in your head to see if you are on pace each lap.

Protocol	**Example for a 16:00 two-mile**
Jog the first lap in goal pace +1:00.	2:00 + 1:00 = 3:00 or 12 minute per mile pace
Jog the second lap in goal pace +:45.	2:00 + :45 = 2:45 or 11 minute per mile pace
Jog the third lap in goal pace +:30.	2:00 + :30 = 2:30 or 10 minute per mile pace
Run the fourth lap in goal pace +:15.	2:00 + :15 = 2:15 or 9 minute per mile pace
Run laps 5 and 6 at goal pace.	2:00 + :00 = 2:00 or 8 minute per mile pace
Run laps 7 and 8 all out as fast and hard as you can.	→

Check your heart monitor every 100 meters during the last two laps. You want to see if your heart rate (HR) has stopped getting higher no matter how much harder and faster you try to run. Remember that you are trying to duplicate the total exhaustion encountered when the treadmill is elevated at the end of a regular stress test. (See the section on the Frank-Starling stall for the rationale behind this format for stress testing.) For some faster runners, the protocol may have to be modified if the 15-second increments increase the pace too quickly.

Again, let me emphasize that these self-tests may not produce the ideal results you could expect if you were tested in a lab following the Balke or Bruce treadmill stress test protocols. Furthermore, hidden coronary artery disease is not going to show up on the HRM, but it probably will during a stress test while your heart is being monitored by an electrocardiogram machine and evaluated by trained personnel. You're on your own out there on the track.

Once you have determined your MHR, just find that number on the inside edge of the right-hand axis of the THR Calculator. You no longer are using your age to predict your max, so ignore the number across from it on the outside of the axis. Draw a line between the number you found and your RHR on the left-hand axis and voila, you'll find your THR numbers where this line intersects the percentage lines. Instant numbers without pain, aka "coach's math."

Anomalies, Paradoxes, and Contradictions in Using a Monitor While Running

As you might appreciate after all that discussion about what you thought was a fairly simple process of setting THR zones, getting started is the hardest part of monitored training. However, please read this section carefully before trying the workouts recommended in the last part of this chapter. Having the wrong numbers for your zones may be bad, but the frustration you'll experience

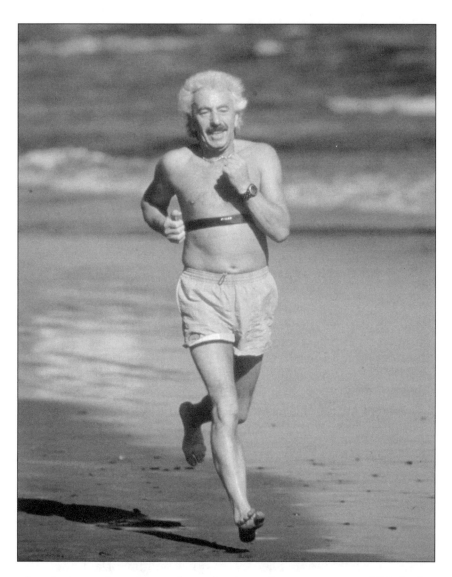

when being a slave to good numbers can be even greater. This is the update that I promised you earlier. This is where exercise cardiology overrules exercise physiology.

The Frank-Starling Stall

Earlier I recommended using a self-test to bring your HR up to maximum over a distance of two miles. That distance (and the time that it takes to run it) actually may be too short. Although it's too complicated for me to explain in great detail here, you do need to understand a little about the Frank-Starling mechanism. It can affect more than just your attempts to reach your MHR.

Coaches Ernest Frank and Otto Starling were exercise physiologists whose work can help us understand today why you can't hit MHR with just one all-out sprint around the track or up a hill. They discovered the fact that the heart's initial response to sudden demand for increased output is to increase stroke volume, not to increase stroke frequency. (Stroke volume is simply the amount of blood that the heart pumps with each beat.) Frank and Starling observed that as the volume of blood in the ventricles increases (up to a certain point), the length of the cardiac muscle fibers increases. This causes more interaction between the heart muscle's fibers, allowing more blood to be forcefully ejected with each beat. This results in a slower-than-expected work rate, modulated by the sinus node, the part of the nervous system that stimulates the cardiac muscle to contract. While this extra time keeps the rate of beats at a lower-than-expected level, it does allow the cardiac output to actually increase. (Cardiac output is the product of stroke volume times stroke frequency.) Therefore, more oxygen-rich blood really is being delivered to the muscle site of the oxygen debt. Monitor users usually find all this hard to believe while seeing illogically low numbers when they feel so dead in their tracks and are huffing and puffing worse than the Little Engine That Could.

Luckily, this phenomenon does not last for long. Just as an increase in running speed is accomplished initially by increasing stride length and then subsequently by increasing the rate of turnover, continued demand for oxygen will be met by increasing the rate of heartbeats. Unfortunately, until this "second wind" arrives, runners encounter a period of woe, agony, pain, and torture. They have to struggle with the dreaded lead leg syndrome, the muscle tightness caused by the quick buildup of lactic acid that follows the muscle's sudden depletion of local oxygen supplies. Once the respiratory and cardiovascular systems have had time to respond with delivery of a fresh supply of oxygen, the expected correlations will return. Your HR, your breathing rate, and your perception of your effort will be back to normal and will make sense. Then, once again, the linear logic of exercise physiology will allow you to train intelligently within the effort zones for your current level of fitness and your general ability, and with a pattern appropriate for your immediate goals.

In summary, the Frank-Starling stall may cause your monitor to stall in your tracks if you take off like a jackrabbit at full speed. If your workout calls for very fast, short repeats of 400 meters or less, or for hard hill work, you may have to set your THR zone several beats lower than you are actually aiming for, or ignore your monitor. Then, over the course of the workout, your HRs should catch up and finish where you would expect them.

Cardiac Creep

You may have noticed that I keep referring to the "linear logic of exercise physiology." I mean, of course, that physiologists expect that changes of effort will result in changes of HR. They have taught us that the harder we run and the harder we huff and puff, the faster our hearts should beat. We know that there is a direct relationship: Go faster to increase HR, slow down to lower HR. But is this always the case?

Well, no. There are times when the path that your working HR takes from resting to maximum is not always a straight (i.e., linear) one, directly correlated with the amount of work that your muscles are doing. Sometimes your heart beats too fast for the pace you're running. This is so because sending oxygen to the muscles is not always the only job that the heart is asked to do. It also works to maintain body temperature. Do these added beats per minute reflect how hard your leg muscles are working? Or only how hard your heart is working? Furthermore, keep in mind that as your blood volume diminishes with the loss of fluid due to sweating, your heart has to beat faster to compensate. Again, your monitor is going to try to convince you that you're working harder.

Well, the good news is that your prime working muscles might not be working harder. Therefore, you may not have to keep slowing down to stay in your effort zone. The surprising fact of the matter is that your heart itself is not getting tired from all this extra "effort." Its energy system is not the same as that of other muscles. It is immune from conventional fatigue and can keep beating at almost maximum for days on end if necessary.

So, how do you accommodate cardiac creep? Well, you start by not being a literal slave to your heart monitor. If your schedule calls for an easy recovery day of jogging at 60–70 percent effort and the weather is warm to hot, give yourself a grace zone of several extra beats per minute. If you are fit enough to normally recover at an

8:00 pace, there is no need to slow down to a walk to avoid going over your target zone. Check the Pace and Effort Chart to see what pace should generate the goal effort for today's workout. Then use some common sense and simply make sure that the workout meets its objective. It should be hard or easy, or sometimes medium.

Before I leave this topic, consider the corollary to the heat. What if it's so cold that your HR stays below 60 percent during a recovery-day workout? Should you crank it up to race pace in an effort to get your HR up into the usual 60–70 percent effort zone? Well, even if your VCR is still blinking "12:00," I hope you're smart enough to stay inside when it's that cold and just bag that workout.

A Few GRIPEs

The last of these paradoxes, contradictions, and anomalies involves the principle of "GRIPEs" (gross responses involving physiological effort), as they are known to many of us coaches. Although we may be sick and tired of hearing our runners complain about why their monitor numbers sometimes don't make sense, our answer probably won't fit under the GRIPE label. The GRIPE principle has us seeing the forest when we may occasionally need to see just a tree or two. In other words, instead of expecting a particular workout to benefit each of the body's working systems equally, perhaps we need to separately evaluate each system's response to yesterday's workload.

For example, when you ask yourself which system—your muscular, your respiratory, or your cardiovascular—worked the hardest during yesterday's workout, you can occasionally explain the unexpected numbers you see on your HRM. I suspect that your lungs, your legs, and your heart may take different amounts of time to recover their energy reserves from a workout. Different workouts may tax these separate systems differently.

Here's an example of what I'm getting at: a long, slow run may leave your leg muscles more exhausted than the respiratory and cardiovascular systems that didn't have to work very hard because the effort was so aerobic. The next day you find your HR surprisingly low despite feeling dead and heavy legged. Feeling so tired, you conclude that you're working quite hard on your recovery run. Paradoxically, when you check your monitor, you see numbers way out of line, far lower than what you expected for the effort you're apparently making. The problem is that you just don't have enough energy back in the leg muscles to allow you to run as hard as you feel you are going. Since, in our minds, slow speed = low numbers = easy effort, we're surprised. So, instead of gross responses, maybe it's a day in which fine, delicate responses are the norm. Give the legs a break, letting them take it so easy that your monitor feels guilty. Ignore the contradiction and be thankful for small favors. Just take it slower than usual and don't feel that you need to apologize to anyone about going so slowly. Today you're listening to your legs instead of your monitor beeper. Remember, miles of smiles are just as important as lots of happy heartbeats.

Don't be a slave to your monitor. You must use it intelligently. The concept of measuring how hard you're working by counting your HR is valid; it is not always 100 percent reliable. In some cases, it will be wiser to stick with your stopwatch as your guide. Other times, neither is worth trusting and you'll have to rely on the common sense of perceived exertion. If what you're doing doesn't feel logical, it might be better to listen to your head than to your heart. Unfortunately, it usually takes a very experienced, veteran runner to know when to do this. In any case, keep in mind that coaches want to see their runners train and race consistently. It's far better, then, to be slightly undertrained than barely over-trained. The health and injury fairies await that latter category of runners with a good case of Inconsistency Disease.

Designing Your Running Program

Now that I've finished preparing you for your Cardiology Med Boards, I'm sure that you'd like an equal amount of advice on how to become a coach. Well, whether you coach yourself or hundreds of runners, choose whichever of the following four basic training patterns is appropriate for your objective. More than one might apply. Be forewarned that the sample training patterns I have included here are just that—samples. Within this one chapter, I can hope to accomplish just one thing: to teach you the value of hard/easy training. The actual workouts that I offer for each day can be modified thousands of ways, so don't get hung up on the details. Just appreciate the suggested training patterns as solid examples of how to put workouts back-to-back so you can stay healthy and yet reach your goal of improved fitness. I am suggesting week-long training patterns to be repeated after each 7-day cycle. There's nothing wrong, however, with changing the length of the cycle to 10 or even 14 days, if you need more recovery time between hard days. Just slip extra easy days into the training pattern so your long-term training is consistent and not disrupted by layoffs from injuries or illness.

You first must decide why you want to use monitored running as your choice of exercise. This is not an easy decision. To get your money's worth from this book, force yourself to read the following material carefully before proceeding to the fun part, that is, the workouts. You will get the maximum benefits from your training with solid preparation.

Your chances of succeeding are greatly improved when you know *why* you are doing something. Review the following list of reasons, goals, or objectives and decide, for each one, whether it applies to you.

1. If you are a beginner seeking the general fitness that helps you stay healthier and better looking, follow the Endurance Training Pattern for Beginning Joggers.

2. If you are a veteran jogger who wants to become a "recreational" runner participating in road races just to finish the distance, but without concern for your finish time or place, start with the Endurance Training Pattern for Runners.

3. If you have been a "competitive" runner training seriously to improve your finish times and places, before you pick a training pattern you must consider several factors: (a) whether you have "peaked" and can't seem to improve, or find that your times are getting slower; (b) whether your workouts have been inconsistent with frequent layoffs due to injuries, illnesses, or other interruptions from life; and (c) whether you have been smart enough to take off for a period of active rest. If any of these things are true of you, then choose the Endurance Training Pattern for Runners for at least six weeks; then move up to the Stamina Training Pattern for Phase II Competitive Runners for the bulk of your racing season.

   If you then want to be assured of peak performances for a short series of races in which you want to be at your all-time, most athletic best, add the Speed Training Pattern for

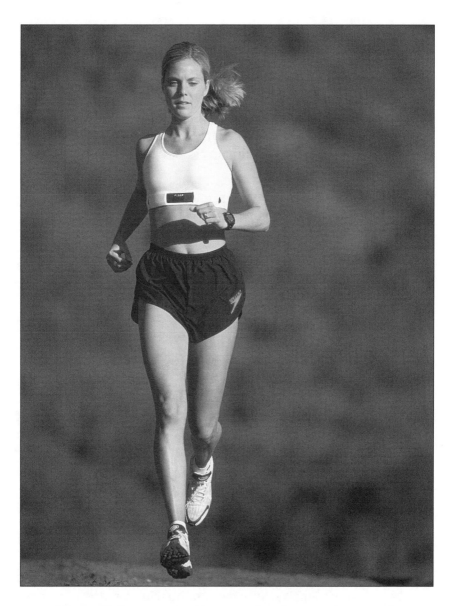

Phase III Competitive Runners for three to four weeks or
until you peak out and your times fall off.

4. If none of the criteria listed apply to you, but your training
has consisted of only "out-the-door" workouts with no
specific guidelines defining the levels of intensity, frequency, or duration for the "hard" or "easy" days of your
training, choose the Stamina Training Pattern for Phase II

Competitive Runners. You can train at this level of intensity for the rest of your life, enjoying both superior health and the option of being a fairly competitive road runner. If you don't like the training pattern because the workouts are too hard or there are too many of them, modify the pattern until you're comfortable. Or just drop down to the Endurance Training Pattern for Runners. At least there is wisdom in following a hard/easy training pattern.

If you are planning to run a marathon, buy a book on that subject after you follow these recommendations to get in great 10K shape. The plans and patterns for marathon training are way beyond the scope of this chapter and, in fact, of most books. In this case you really should find a private coach who will design your own personal program.

Adjusting Intensity in Your Running Workouts

The following running programs are based on daily patterns of workouts that are repeated from week to week. Changes in intensity will occur from day to day within a weekly pattern in compliance with the Hard/Easy principle of exercise physiology: stress followed by recovery allows adaptation. Workout intensity will also change from pattern to pattern and will take the shape of the pyramid, which coaches affectionately call a "Training Triangle." The easier workouts of lower intensity form the base of the triangle. As a runner's goals change, the patterns change so the separate components of fitness (endurance, stamina, speed) can be developed, in sequence, one building block on top of another. As the intensity increases on the trip up to the top of the triangle, the total distance of the workouts is decreased in order to keep the runner from overtraining. Thus, the shape of the pyramid illustrates how a competitive runner can reach a "peak" performance.

TRAINING PLAN

ENDURANCE TRAINING PATTERN FOR BEGINNING JOGGERS

This will be the ideal training pattern to develop endurance for beginning joggers. It is also the pattern that advanced, competitive runners follow when they rebuild their aerobic base at the start of each season.

First, a caveat: You must be careful here. You don't want to get hurt trying to go too far too soon. Please be a patient Republican and stick with this conservative pattern. It may take from 6 to 12 weeks or even longer to graduate to the next pattern, so be patient. The objective is to get you fit enough to jog anywhere you want to go.

EASY DAYS: MONDAYS, WEDNESDAYS, AND FRIDAYS

Move along at a comfortable pace equal to a "stroll." Do not try marching fast! Racewalking or marching can be more biomechanically stressful than jogging or running.

Walk for 20 to 30 minutes to elevate your HR to at least 20 beats per minute above your RHR but without exceeding 60 percent effort as indicated on the THR Calculator. Your THR zone will be ____to____beats per minute. (Look up the numbers and fill them in.) Set your monitor for that zone, and if you approach 60 percent, slow down your pace.

HARD DAYS: TUESDAYS AND THURSDAYS

Stroll for 5 minutes to warm up. Then imagine taking your heart for a ride on a roller coaster. You want your HR to climb to the higher end of your target zone and then drop back down to the lower end of your zone.

Start jogging until you hit 75 percent effort. Then walk until you have recovered down to 60 percent effort. Keep repeating this pattern until you have covered 15–20 minutes. If your leg muscles tighten up, walk the rest of the workout to avoid the dreaded shinsplints or muscle cramps. Your THR zone is ____to____beats per minute.

Stroll another 5 minutes as a cool-down.

LONG, HARD DAY: SATURDAYS OR SUNDAYS

Pick one of these traditional days for your weekly long workout. Take off the other day and enjoy life. Even though the intensity is low, this workout qualifies as a hard day because of its length.

Walk for 10–20 minutes without exceeding 60 percent. Then jog/walk for 15-20 minutes at your hard-day 75 percent to 60 percent up-and-down effort zone. Finish with another 10–20-minute walk at less than 60 percent.

Keep repeating this weekly training pattern until you can jog all the workouts without walking or exceeding 75 percent effort. The goal is to develop your cardiovascular and muscular endurance so your muscles can keep repeating the jogging movement through that specific range of motion without fatiguing and quitting before you reach your goal destination.

I have designed a six-day pattern that you may find too difficult or ambitious. In that case, skip one or some or all of the easy days. When you want to be fitter and better looking, just add in the easy days. If you are already jogging all of your hard-day workouts, start with jog/walk easy days and slowly fill them with all-jogging workouts. You then, if you wish, will be ready for a slightly harder training pattern like the one that follows.

TRAINING PLAN

ENDURANCE TRAINING PATTERN FOR RUNNERS

This training pattern will serve as phase I of the four traditional conditioning cycles that competitive runners must experience to develop their full athletic potential. This phase will develop "aerobic conditioning." It can also serve beginning joggers seeking a little higher level of fitness, good looks, and more endurance once they have completed their first pattern.

EASY DAYS: MONDAYS, WEDNESDAYS, AND FRIDAYS

Since these must be recovery days, they have to be slow to the point where they may be biomechanically uncomfortable. Too bad! Just trust your monitor and cool it. You will grow accustomed to this slower pace. After your workouts, you can loosen up with stretching and several "strides," those short (about 10–15 seconds), smooth, but fast runs that you see the elite runners doing to loosen up at the start of a race.

Jog 30–45 minutes at 60–70 percent effort. Your THR zone is ____to____beats per minute. If the weather is warm or hot, see the earlier discussion of cardiac creep. And make sure you stretch and run four to six strides after you finish your recovery jog. It's very important to undo the bad biomechanical side effects of slow jogging that eventually cause weakness and tightness in your legs. Stretch and stride your way to young legs!

HARD DAYS: TUESDAYS AND SATURDAYS

Warm up for 5–10 minutes with easy jogging. Then stretch and run a few strides.

Run 15–30 minutes of Heart Rate Fartlek. This is the modern day version of the "speed play" (translation for "fartlek") workouts invented by the Swedes in the 1940s. Running this workout using the telemetric HRM first developed by the Finns may make you an Honorary Scandinavian! Just follow the same "roller-coaster" pattern as described earlier for beginner joggers. Set your THR zone at 65–75 percent effort at ____to____beats per minute if the weather is cool or at 70–80 percent effort at ____to____beats per minute if it's warm or hot. Enjoy some "speed" work as you run faster to elevate your HR to the upper zone limit. When your monitor beeps at your upper limit, hit the brakes and jog slowly until it beeps again at your lower limit.

Jog for 5:00 to cool down.

MODERATE DAY: THURSDAYS

This is a simple, straightforward run. Just ease down the road for several minutes at warm-up pace and effort.

Once you're warm and sweating, pick up the pace until you reach your steady state effort of 75–80 percent. Your THR is ____to____beats per minute. Enjoy running comfortably for 20–40 minutes.

Don't forget to cool down for 5 minutes.

HARD, LONG DAY: SUNDAYS

Experience had taught me, long before I discovered the reasons for cardiac creep, to allow an extra 5 percent margin for long runs. That's why you'll have a very generous 15 percent range of effort for this workout.

Set your monitor at 60–75 percent of your maximal effort. Your THR zone is ____to____beats per minute. Run easily for 45 to 60 minutes.

Avoid the temptation to push the effort up into the 70–75 percent zone right away. Save that extra 5 percent for the last part of the workout when you'll be a bit dehydrated and the monitor might be suggesting that you slow down. If you feel tired, and your HR is at 75 percent, you will have to back off the pace and keep that monitor from beeping.

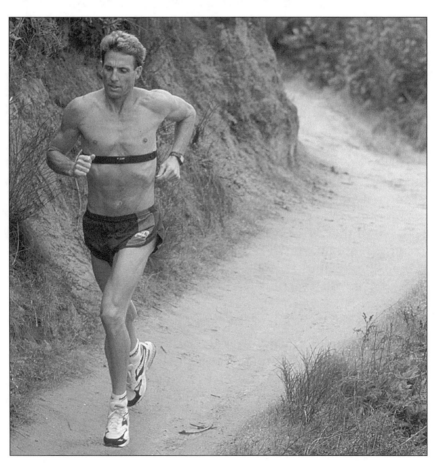

TRAINING PLAN

ENDURANCE TRAINING PATTERN FOR RUNNERS

To me, stamina is the ability to maintain the goal pace during a run or race without slowing down very much. It is the next higher level of fitness above endurance. Phase II workouts will concentrate on improving your "anaerobic conditioning," that is, your ability to huff and puff and not get too tired. Follow this training pattern for four weeks. Then, if you are a competitive runner, run a race to see what kind of shape you're in after all this preparation.

EASY DAYS: MONDAYS, WEDNESDAYS, AND FRIDAYS

Follow the same pattern of workouts that you used for endurance training in phase I. With the hard days getting harder, these easy days take on even more importance. You may have to cut back on the length of your runs in order to ensure recovery. Be sure to stretch and run some strides after you finish the run to compensate for the slow pace.

Set your monitor at 60–70 percent effort. Your THRs are ____to____beats per minute. And don't forget to stretch and run your strides before you head for the shower.

HARD DAY: TUESDAYS

Go to a track and do the usual warm-up of jogging, stretching, and striding to get ready for a real interval workout.

Run one mile three times at 80–85 percent effort with a 400-meter recovery jog between each separate mile to allow your HR to return to at least 70 percent before starting the next mile. Your THRs are ____to____beats per minute during the repeat miles and ____beats per minute at the end of the 400-meter recovery interval.

Jog 5:00 to cool down.

HARD DAY: THURSDAYS

Warm up by jogging at 60–70 percent effort until you are sweating. Then pick up the pace for 4 or 5 minutes to 75–80 percent.

Next, increase your effort to 85 percent and run at this approximate lactate threshold for 15 minutes. Cool down by jogging for another 5:00. Since this workout covers such a wide range of effort, just focus on the important lactate threshold part by setting your monitor at 80–85 percent. Your THRs are ____to____beats per minute.

HARD DAY: SATURDAYS

Try to find a hilly route where you can enjoy a Heart Rate Fartlek workout with the hills supplying the effort required to elevate your HR. If you're a flatlander, you'll simply have to push the pace fast enough to hit 85 percent. Whether on hills or flats, once you reach 85 percent, slow down to recover to 70 percent. If you hit 85 percent before reaching the top of the hill, start slowing down right there. And, obviously, if you haven't hit 85 percent by the top of the hill, *do not* try sprinting down the other side of the hill to reach 85 percent. The idea is to work within the 70–85 percent effort range with a series of pace changes. The Swedes defined their word *fartlek* as "speed play" and offered it as a creative option to the regimentation of interval workouts on the track. Your THRs at 70–85 percent are ____to____beats per minute.
    Jog at 60 percent for 5:00 to cool down.

MODERATE DAY: SUNDAYS

Your weekly long run now has to take on the primary job of allowing you to recover from these three ambitiously hard workouts. Lower your upper THR zone limit to 70 percent and shorten the length of the run, if necessary, to guarantee recovery. Be sure to stretch and run some strides before heading for the shower. Your THRs at 60–70 percent are ____to____beats per minute.

TRAINING PLAN

SPEED TRAINING PATTERN FOR PHASE III COMPETITIVE RUNNERS

I define "speed" for runners as the ability to run faster than race pace. To assure that race pace feels relaxing and not like top speed, the featured workouts in phase III are run faster than goal pace, but not necessarily at top, or sprint, speed. Notice here that I have referred exclusively to pace in this discussion. It's now time to fully utilize EBT.

Since you ended phase II with a 5K or 10K race, it's time to correlate your HRs with your minutes per mile workout paces. Check table 4.1 to find your race time in the second or third column from the left side. Along that horizontal line under your time, as you read to the right, will be your suggested workout paces. I'll supply the percentages of effort for each type of workout, and you'll have to look up the expected pace on the chart.

EASY DAYS: MONDAYS, WEDNESDAYS, AND FRIDAYS

Take one or two of these days completely off to ensure freshness and recovery so the hard days can really be fast. If you need the mileage, don't go too far. You do, however, need to lower the upper limit to guarantee that the carbos you eat can be converted into glycogen and stored up for the next hard day. By your staying so aerobic, the main source of energy will be fats, allowing the glycogen to be spared.

Jog at 60–65 percent effort for 30–45 minutes with your monitor set at ____to____beats per minute. Your pace should be ___minutes per mile.

Stretch and run five to six strides for 15 seconds.

HARD DAY: TUESDAYS

After the usual warm-up activities at the track, do the following speed workout.

Run 400 meters 10–12 times in ____(fill in your time) at 90–95 percent effort with a slow 200-meter recovery jog between each 400 meters. Your THRs at the end of the 400-meter repeats will be ____to____beats per minute. At the end of your 200-meter recovery jog, your HR should be at least ____beats per minute or lower.

Jog 5:00 to cool down.

HARD DAY: THURSDAYS

If you have a race coming up this weekend, just do one-half to one-third of this workout. Warm up as usual.

Do a lactate threshold run of 20 minutes according to the instructions for phase II as given earlier. Your pace should be __:__minutes per mile, and your THRs will be ____to____beats per minute. Don't forget to cool down.

HARD DAY: SATURDAYS

If you are not racing, repeat Saturday's phase II workout of Heart Rate Fartlek. Since this is a variable-speed workout, there are no pace per mile recommendations. Your THR zone will be ____to____beats per minute.

Jog at 60 percent to cool down for 5 minutes.

RECOVERY DAY: SUNDAYS

Shorten this run to just 30 minutes and use the same criteria as for the phase II Sunday run. Your pace should be __:__per mile, and your THRs at 60–70 percent will be ____to____beats per minute.

Stretch and stride as your cool-down.

In Summary: The Long (Hard) and Short (Easy) of It

Effort-based training consists of measuring workout quality with beats per minute plus minutes per mile plus common sense. Once you've selected valid THRs, know what kind of shape you're in, and appreciate how closely HR and pace are correlated, you are on the road to smart training. Although I've given you some reasons to take your HRM readings with a grain of salt, I haven't given you license to ignore common sense. It all boils down to following the greatest principle of training: hard/easy.

Don't race your workouts in order to be a "workout winner," and don't push it on your easy days. Frequent, moderate workouts done on a consistent basis are the real secret to good health and fast times. Let's see if you can train smart enough to be the oldest, healthiest person to ever die.

Carpe ventum!

CHAPTER 5

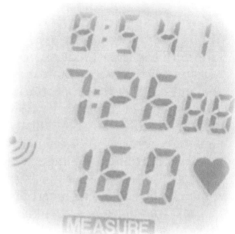

CYCLING

JOE FRIEL

In his first year as an Expert-level mountain bike racer, Chad Matteson was disappointed with his results. In eight races, his best finish was 13th, but he was usually much farther back. He even failed to finish three races. The following winter, Matteson, a 24-year-old college student from Colorado Springs, Colorado, started training in a new way—with a heart rate monitor. In the next season, despite suffering a dislocated shoulder in a racing crash in early June, he accumulated six wins in the Expert division and several top-five placements. At the end of the season he upgraded to the Elite category, finishing 7th in his first Elite/Pro race. Matteson's dramatic turnaround was largely due to learning how to train and race on the basis of his heart rate.

While you may not experience such remarkable changes in fitness, if you've never used one before there is little doubt that knowing how to train with a heart rate monitor can give your cycling a boost. Whether you race, do century rides, or ride strictly for fitness, monitoring heart rate can help you improve.

Using Heart Rate Monitoring for Cycling

Within each workout are two important elements. The first is duration—the time or distance of the ride. Duration is easy to measure with a stopwatch or handlebar computer. The other element, and generally the more important, is intensity. In the past, athletes gauged intensity by how they felt. While perception of intensity is still a valuable skill, it can be inaccurate due to excitement or varying levels of motivation. Now, with a heart rate monitor, controlling the intensity of a workout is quite precise.

Heart rate training for cycling is based on the use of specific training zones to achieve certain benefits. Once you know your personal training zones, reaping the physiological rewards of any workout is easy. This method takes the guesswork out of training.

There are five training benefits that come from staying within certain heart rate zones during workouts. They are listed here from the lowest to the highest intensity.

- **Active recovery.** Easy rides, when done by well-conditioned athletes, speed up the recovery process by opening capillaries and sending fresh blood through the muscles to remove waste products and bring in oxygen and carbohydrates. These rides typically follow a race or other high-intensity workout. The active-recovery intensity is also often used as the rest period in interval-type workouts and as warm-up and cool-down.

- **Aerobic endurance.** This benefit is fundamental to aerobic fitness regardless of your reason for riding. It includes a strengthened heart, efficient central nervous system, increased capillary beds within working muscles, improved oxygen uptake capabilities, and elevated utilization of fat for fuel while precious glycogen is spared. This intensity also gets you used to being on the bike for long periods.

- **Lactate threshold.** Improved speed, comfort, and endurance at or near lactate threshold effort is a tremendous benefit and is highly trainable. Lactate threshold is the level of intensity at which lactate, an acidic by-product of exercise, accumulates in the blood. By improving lactate

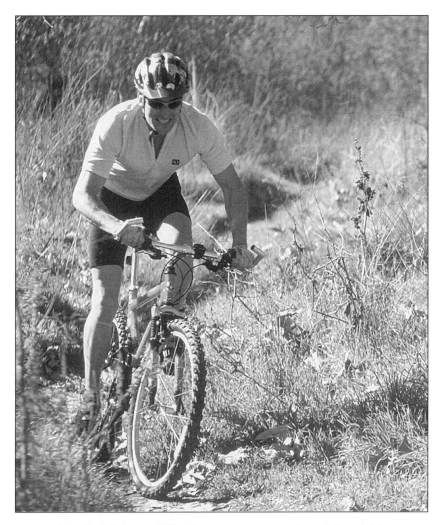

threshold, you will be faster, more comfortable, and better able to maintain efforts near this intensity. Lactate threshold is sometimes called "anaerobic threshold."

- **Aerobic capacity.** This benefit includes a boosted ability to deliver and use oxygen for the production of energy. Also improved at this intensity is economy—the ability to pedal smoothly and waste little energy while near maximum effort for an extended time as in a long sprint or fast hill climb.

- **Anaerobic capacity.** This is the ability to create muscular power at near maximal levels for short periods, such as in sprints of less than 20 seconds.

Finding Your Optimal Training Intensity for Cycling

In order to achieve these benefits, you must train at specific heart rate zones based on a reference point unique to your physiology. Maximal heart rate is a commonly used reference, but another and potentially more accurate method is to base training zones on lactate threshold heart rate (LTHR). The reason has to do with individualizing the zones. For example, if we took a cross section of riders of different abilities and ages, but all having the same maximal heart rate, we'd find that their LTHRs varied by several beats. If you reference training zones to LTHR, training is more individualized to your unique needs.

The problem with this method is in initially estimating LTHR. Some racers have a sense of their LTHR from observing their heart rate monitors when the feelings of lactate become apparent in races and hard rides. For others, and for most experienced riders, a test is necessary.

I have developed two simple tests to estimate LTHR for the cyclists I train.

Lactate Threshold Test on Trainer

The first test is a variation of the Conconi test and involves the use of an indoor training device and a handlebar computer that picks up speed from the rear wheel. A CompuTrainer, Cateye CS-1000 Cyclosimulator, or Cycle Ops Electronic Trainer may also be used. You will need an assistant; a bike with a rear-wheel computer pickup; and a magnetic, fluid, or wind-load trainer with a high load potential. Warm up for 10 minutes, and then follow these steps:

1. Start at 15 miles per hour. Every minute, increase speed by 1 mile per hour by pedaling faster or by shifting. Do not stand during the test.

2. At the end of each minute, the assistant records your heart rate and rating of perceived exertion (RPE) based on table 5.1.

TABLE 5.1	Rating of Perceived Exertion (RPE) Scale

RPE	Description
6	No exertion at all
7	Extremely light
8	
9	Very light
10	
11	Light
12	
13	Somewhat hard
14	
15	Hard (heavy)
16	
17	Very hard
18	
19	Extremely hard
20	Maximal exertion

Borg RPE Scale © Gunnar Borg, 1970, 1985, 1994, 1998.
G. Borg, 1998, *Borg's Perceived Exertion and Pain Scales* (Champaign, IL: Human Kinetics) p. 47.

3. Continue increasing speed and recording data in this way until you can no longer maintain speed.

4. Your assistant should listen closely to your breathing to detect when it becomes labored and should place a "VT" (ventilatory threshold) on the data sheet next to the appropriate stage when this occurs.

5. The data collected should look something like the data in table 5.2.

→

TABLE 5.2	Lactate Threshold Test Example		
Speed	Heart rate	RPE	
15	110	8	
16	118	10	
17	125	12	
18	135	13	
19	142	14	
20	147	15	
21	153	17	VT
22	156	19	
23	159	20	

6. Compare VT heart rate with an exertion rating of 15–17 to determine LTHR. If VT falls below this range, use heart rate at 15 RPE as LTHR. If VT is above the range of 15–17, use heart rate at 17 RPE as LTHR.

Individual Time-Trial Lactate Threshold Test

The second test I use to estimate LTHR for my clients is based on completing an individual time trial, either in a race or as a workout. Wear your heart rate monitor and start it with your time-trial start. Stop it as you cross the finish line, and later recall the average heart rate for the ride. Use table 5.3 to estimate your LTHR.

In order to get an accurate LTHR, you may need to repeat the test on another day, always waiting until you're fully

TABLE 5.3	Lactate Threshold Heart Rate Estimated From Individual Time Trial

Divide average heart rate from time trial by number in appropriate column based on event distance. The result is your estimated LTHR.

Distance of time trial	Done as race	Done as workout
5K	1.10	1.04
10K	1.07	1.02
8–10 mi.	1.05	1.01
40K	1.00	0.97

recovered, or to perform the two tests on two different days. The more times you complete the tests, the more accurate your LTHR estimate will become.

Once you have estimated LTHR, you can determine training zones from table 5.4. By training in these heart rate zones, you'll reap the benefits listed in the right-hand column.

TABLE 5.4	Heart Rate Training Zones as Percent of Lactate Threshold Heart Rate (LTHR)

Zone	Percent of LTHR	Workout type	Benefit
1	65–81	Short duration	Active recovery
2	82–88	Long duration	Extensive aerobic endurance
3	89–93	Medium duration	Intensive aerobic endurance
4	94–99	Intervals/tempo	Lactate threshold
5a	100–102	Intervals/tempo	Lactate threshold
5b	103–105	Intervals	Aerobic capacity
5c	106+	Sprints	Anaerobic capacity

The only exception to heart rate training from this table is for zone 5c. During working out to improve anaerobic capacity, the sprints are too short for the heart rate monitor to register quickly enough. With explosive efforts lasting only a few seconds, the heart rate does not have enough time to reach a stable level. A perceived maximal effort is necessary in this case. For all other zones, however, your heart rate monitor will keep you on track.

Designing Your Cycling Program

Using training zones, you should now be able to gauge the intensity of your rides. Of course, it's also necessary to know how the workouts for these zones should be organized and to know the best way to blend them during a week to improve your fitness. This section will show you how to do both.

The following are suggested workouts for each of the zones listed in table 5.4. The durations of these zone-specific workouts are intended for those who typically train 8 to 12 hours in a week. Novice riders who train less than that should reduce the duration accordingly, and those who ride more than about 12 weekly hours may want to increase their duration.

Zone 1—Active Recovery

Ride for one to two hours on a mostly flat course. Use the small chain ring only. If you're new to cycling, taking the day off rather than riding easily is better for speeding your recovery.

Zone 2—Aerobic Endurance

These are rides of at least one hour in which the first few minutes, perhaps 10 to 20, are in zone 1 as a warm-up. Then stay primarily in zone 2 until starting to cool down the last 5 to 10 minutes, again in zone 1. At first, the small chain ring may bring you to zone 2, but later, as fitness improves, the large chain ring will be necessary.

The course should be rolling, in other words, should have gradual hills that take less than two minutes to ascend and don't require you to reduce cadence by more than 10 revolutions per minute. Stay in the saddle on these hills to build greater hip extension strength. Approximately half of your weekly riding time is in this zone.

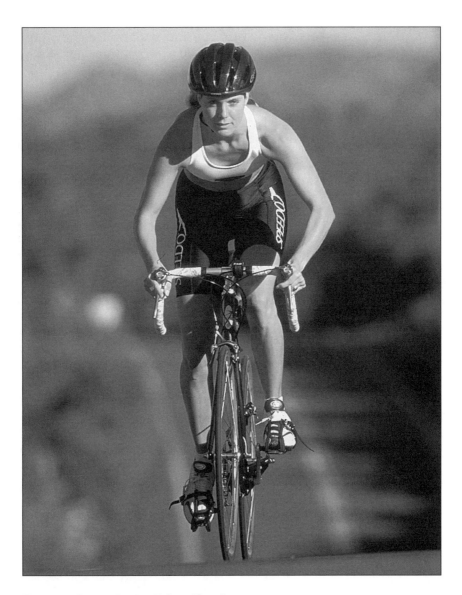

Zone 3—Aerobic Endurance

This higher aerobic endurance intensity brings many of the same benefits as zone 2, but more rapidly depletes carbohydrates while placing moderate stress on the mechanisms of lactate threshold. Zone 3 stress is inadequate to create high levels of fitness but requires recovery time, so it is of limited value. Most riders spend too much time in this zone.

Early in the seasonal preparation period, usually in early winter, continuous rides in this zone may last 20 to 60 minutes, depending on your experience. Long efforts in this zone are done as "controlled" time-trial-type rides on mostly flat courses in the large chain ring. Once a base of aerobic endurance is established, this zone should be avoided by the competitive athlete and used infrequently by the recreational rider.

Zones 4 and 5a—Lactate Threshold

These zones are quite effective in improving fitness without the risk of overtraining or injury associated with the higher zones. They may also be used throughout the year. Early in the training season, while you are still building aerobic fitness, use zone 4. Later in the season, once aerobic endurance is well established, concentrate more on zone 5a. Just as with the zone 3 workouts, ride on mostly flat courses in the large chain ring.

There are two types of lactate threshold workouts. The first is called "cruise intervals" and involves doing 6 to 12 minutes, three to five times, with 2- to 3-minute recoveries after each one (for example, 6 minutes three times, with 2-minute rest breaks). The work interval starts as soon as you begin to apply high force to the pedal. Heart rate should rise into the appropriate zone in the first minute or so. Highly experienced and fit athletes may do up to three repeats that are as long as 20 minutes each with 5-minute recoveries. Cruise intervals may be done on steady uphills to increase power while developing lactate threshold.

The second lactate threshold workout is called "tempo" and is simply a continuous effort lasting 15 to 40 minutes within zones 4 and 5a. This will feel much like a time trial, and besides improving lactate threshold, will enhance your ability to concentrate. Do this workout only after you have completed several weeks of cruise intervals.

Zone 5b—Aerobic Capacity

The benefits of training at this intensity are great for the competitive racer, since this is the intensity associated with the critical moments in races—frequent high speeds, breakaways, climbs, and bridging attempts. Riders who do not race have less need for this type of training but may do it for variety, as a challenge, or to attain higher fitness levels.

Zone 5b workouts come with a great expense. Riding at this level, and higher, places great stress on the body and puts you at risk for overtraining. Active-recovery days are definitely needed following a 5b workout.

Aerobic capacity training involves completing three to five work intervals that are two to five minutes long. The work interval begins as soon as you begin to ride hard. Recover after each one for the same length of time it took to do the preceding interval. For example, do four minutes three times with four-minute recoveries. These may also be done on a hill to stimulate power development. Heart rate should rise into the 5b zone on each repetition.

Zone 5c—Anaerobic Capacity

These workouts develop the explosive power necessary for intense but short sprints that often determine the outcomes of races. To develop such power, do three sets of five to eight sprints of 8–15 seconds' duration at maximal effort. These can be done on a flat road in a high gear, or up a hill. Recover for a minute between sprints and for five minutes between sets. If you find it difficult to produce maximal effort before you've completed a set, either allow more recovery time both between sprints and between sets, or reduce the number of sprints within a set. It does you no good to practice sprinting at less than top effort.

It's essential that you warm up well before such a session. Complete a few of these workouts by yourself to perfect your sprinting technique before doing them with other riders. These sprints are too short for your heart rate monitor to provide feedback. Do them strictly by perceived effort.

Adjusting Intensity in Your Cycling Workouts

The workouts I have described are like the pieces of a puzzle; they mean nothing until you put them together in a meaningful pattern. Training patterns are usually arranged around seven-day periods, since that model best fits most lifestyles. The types of workouts and the days on which you assign them depend on what your training purpose is.

Fitness Cycling

For the recreational rider who wants to use a bicycle to improve general fitness and burn calories, the most common workouts are those for zones 2 and 3 with a little zone 4 and 5a included. Here is a suggested week for such a rider. All workout durations include warm-up and cool-down in zone 1.

TRAINING PLAN

Monday	Day off
Tuesday	Bike 30–60 minutes including zone 3
Wednesday	Cross-train 30–60 minutes
Thursday	Bike 30–60 minutes including zones 4 and 5a
Friday	Day off
Saturday	Cross-train 45–75 minutes
Sunday	Bike 60–90 minutes including zone 2

Century Training

Once a rider has completed a 100-mile ("century") ride, thoughts invariably turn to how fast it can be done the next time. Other than riding with a group, the best way to improve on your century time is to elevate your lactate threshold. The following suggested week assumes that you have built an endurance base with 8 to 12 weeks of zone 2 and 3 training before starting this schedule. An additional 8 to 12 weeks of such training will bring you to a peak for a fast century. Listed here are suggested bike workouts for "buildup" weeks and rest weeks. Follow the rest-week pattern every fourth week to allow your body to "absorb" the stresses of the previous three weeks and gain fitness. The week of the century is a rest week. As far as the length of the workout goes, start from where you are when beginning this schedule and slowly progress in 10 percent increments to the longer durations. Workout durations include warm-up and cool-down time.

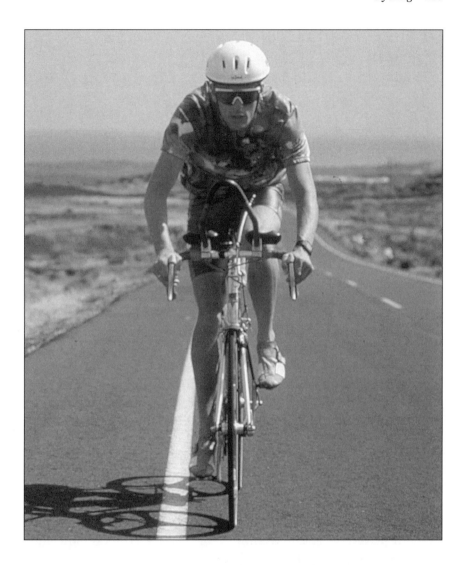

TRAINING PLAN

BUILDUP WEEK

Monday	Day off
Tuesday	1–2 hours, zones 4–5a
Wednesday	1 hour, zone 1
Thursday	1–2 hours, zones 4–5a

Friday	1 hour, zone 1
Saturday	1–2 hours, zone 2
Sunday	2–5 hours, zone 2

REST WEEK

Monday	Day off
Tuesday	1 hour, zone 2
Wednesday	1 hour, zone 3
Thursday	1 hour, zone 1
Friday	Day off
Saturday	1 hour, zone 2
Sunday	1.5–2.5 hours, zone 2

Racing

The cyclist who races employs a broad spectrum of zone-based workouts and has a complex schedule because of the need to create fitness for many different situations from individual time trials to sprints to climbs. To make matters worse, cycling races vary from 45-minute criteriums with an emphasis on sprint speed to 120-mile road races requiring great endurance. Cycling, with its mix of physiological abilities, is one of the most complicated endurance sports for which to train.

The following suggested schedule is designed for the athlete who primarily competes in criteriums and three-hour road races. Training for longer races will necessitate greater training volumes than proposed here. The training year has been divided into four periods—base, build, peak, and race.

Base-Period Training

"Base" is the period during which the rider creates great aerobic endurance, strength, and lactate threshold fitness; it generally occurs in the early-winter months of November through January. Riders in the northern range of states may find it necessary to frequently train indoors. I tell the riders I train that when they are forced indoors for the third consecutive time, they should cross-train instead of riding on a trainer. Too much indoor training leads to burnout. By the end of this period, training volume should be at a high point for the season. It may be necessary to return to the base period later in the year following a period of inactivity due to travel or other conflicts, or even after an extended period of reduced training during the race period. The following is a typical base week. After three such weeks, two if you have difficulty recovering, reduce the training volume by 40 percent for a week to rest and recharge your batteries.

Throughout the season, the racer must continue working to perfect pedaling speed and sprint technique. Much of this is accomplished with "form sprints." These involve doing one sprint of about eight seconds every five minutes. Five to eight such form sprints are best done on a slightly downhill section of road or with a tailwind to keep the heart rate and effort low but to maximize leg turnover. Practice sprinting seated, standing, and mixing the two.

TRAINING PLAN

BASE WEEK

Monday	Day off
Tuesday	1–2 hours, zones 2–3, including form sprints
Wednesday	1–2 hours, zones 4–5a
Thursday	1 hour, zone 1
Friday	1–2 hours, zone 2
Saturday	2–3 hours, zones 4–5, hills
Sunday	3–4 hours, zone 2

Build-Period Training

In the "build" period, the racer reduces training volume and places greater emphasis on anaerobic training in zones 4 through 5c. I suggest two build periods within a season. The first is generally eight weeks long and is planned for the winter months of February and March as you get ready for the first high-priority races in late April and May. After this period of racing, returning to the build period for another four to six weeks will get you ready for the late-season races.

In the build period, endurance is maintained with a weekly, long zone 2 ride. Typically low-priority races are scheduled at this time, and group rides take on the characteristics of races. One of the high-intensity workouts (zones 5b–5c) should be in the hills to continue developing climbing strength. This is the period when you are most likely to overtrain because of the frequent high-intensity work. It's important to keep the recovery days no higher than zone 1 or to take these days off. Prevention is the best way to deal with overtraining. As with the base period, every fourth week should be for rest with reduced volume and intensity.

TRAINING PLAN

BUILD WEEK

Monday	Day off
Tuesday	1–2 hours, zone 5c, may be on hills
Wednesday	1–2 hours, zone 1
Thursday	1–2 hours, zone 5b; may be on hills
Friday	1 hour, zone 1
Saturday	2 hours, all zones, group ride or low-priority race
Sunday	3 hours, zone 1–2 mixed

Peak-Period Training

The peak period is a time of transition between the high intensity of the build period and the race period, when the elements of fitness must all come together. About two weeks are adequate following a build period for producing race fitness. Weekly volume is further reduced, and the training emphasis is put on simulating race intensity and fully recovering between these difficult workouts. While there are fewer hard workouts in this phase of training, those workouts should challenge you. One tune-up race or race-intensity group ride should be done on each weekend.

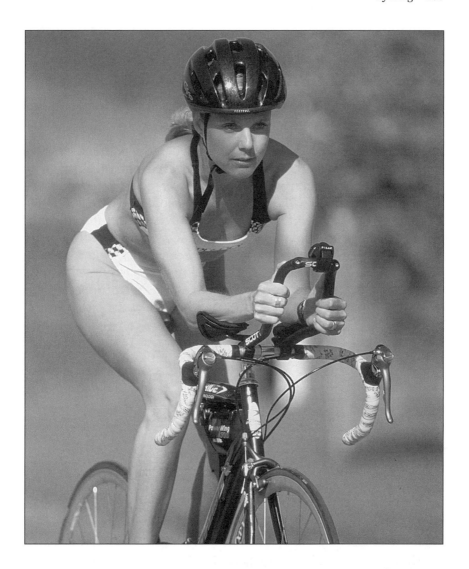

TRAINING PLAN

PEAK WEEK

Monday	Day off
Tuesday	1–2 hours, zone 2, form sprints
Wednesday	1–2 hours, zones 5b–5c; may be on hills
Thursday	1 hour, zone 1

Friday	1 hour, zone 2, form sprints
Saturday	1.5–3 hours, all zones, race or group ride
Sunday	2–3 hours, zones 1–2 mixed

Race-Period Training

During the race period, training volume is reduced once again to ensure that you're rested and ready for the weekend races that now serve as zone 5b and 5c workouts. At midweek, lactate threshold fitness is maintained with a zone 4–5a workout. This is a good time to practice time trialing in the aero position to prepare for time-trial races. Form sprints maintain high-cadence pedaling techniques.

The race period may last as long as six weeks. Trying to stretch it beyond that will often bring diminishing race results as fitness erodes. The better your aerobic fitness established during the base period, the longer you can maintain your race fitness. After the first race period of the season, it's usually a good idea to take a one- to two-week break from training before going back to the base or the build period. This helps to prevent burnout later in the season when you are preparing for a second race period.

TRAINING PLAN

RACE WEEK

Monday	Day off
Tuesday	1–2 hours, zone 2, form sprints
Wednesday	1–2 hours, zones 4–5a; may be on hills
Thursday	1 hour, zone 1
Friday	1 hour, zone 2, form sprints
Saturday	1.5–3 hours, all zones, race or group ride
Sunday	1.5–2 hours, zone 1

Measuring Progress

In the back of every rider's head, from the novice to the most serious racer, is the burning question: Am I improving? The heart rate monitor makes answering that question easy, even when there aren't races or other indicators to use as standards. Simple tests based on the relationship between work output and heart rate provide the answer.

We know that when aerobic fitness improves, as it must in order for a rider to improve as an endurance cyclist, heart rate goes down for any given level of work as measured by speed or power. In the same way, when heart rate remains constant, the work output of a rider will increase as aerobic fitness improves. There are two simple self-tests using these principles that you can do to check progress. First, you can simply repeat the LTHR test on an indoor trainer as discussed earlier in this chapter. Create an x-y graph with speed as a constant on the horizontal axis and heart rate as the variable on the vertical axis. A shift of the graphed line to the right on retests shows positive proof of improving aerobic fitness. Figure 5.1 illustrates this.

I call my other self-test an "aerobic time trial." Find a flat two- or three-mile course with no stop signs and low traffic. You'll ride this route as an out-and-back course, making it a four- to six-mile total test distance. Mark or use fixed landmarks at the start/finish and turnaround points for subsequent tests. Warm up for 10 to 20

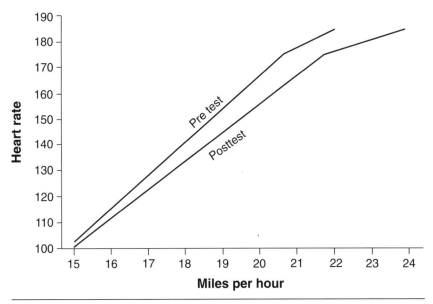

Figure 5.1 Lactate threshold heart rate tests before and after a period of training. Fitness improvement is evident from the shift to the right of the posttest.

minutes, gradually bringing your heart up to zone 4. Once you have attained a heart rate 10 beats below your LTHR, ride the course staying within 1 beat of that heart rate. Time yourself. A faster time indicates improving fitness.

If you've been training for three or more years, don't expect big changes in your self-test results. A change of 2 percent is significant when you're already in great shape.

Breaking Away

Gone are the days of training by the seat of the pants and guessing how you're doing. The heart rate monitor has forever changed the way we get in shape for cycling. You have on your wrist the basis for a personal fitness revolution of greater magnitude than all the discoveries of exercise science in this century. If you've never owned a heart rate monitor before, or if you had one but didn't know how to use it, you're in for an exciting change. By merely determining your unique training zones and intelligently training with them to achieve specific benefits, you have greater cycling fitness at your fingertips.

CHAPTER 6

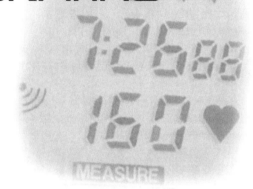

IN-LINE SKATING

FRANK J. FEDEL

In-line skating offers benefits not available from any other activity. Leg muscles are developed in a unique way, the cardiovascular system is challenged, and the impact-free nature of in-line skating makes it ideal for anyone looking for an alternative to most mainstream activities.

In terms of muscle use during in-line skating, the well-rounded hip muscle development that occurs as a result of the lateral motion of the legs cannot be achieved with conventional cardiovascular sports. Thigh and gluteal muscle development is a natural response to the repetitive "semi-static" bent-knee position that occurs during the glide phase (just before the push-off phase) of each stride during skating. And the bent-over position adopted by skaters traveling faster than 14–15 miles per hour places your trunk in a position similar to that taken during cycling—making in-line skating a somewhat familiar-feeling exercise for cyclists. Of course, whereas with cycling you are supported by your arms, there is no support for your upper body with in-line skating; therefore the lower back is also exercised during in-line skating.

Although many similarities exist between the movements that occur during in-line skating, running, and cycling, in-line skating offers some advantages. During cycling, you are supported by a bicycle seat; during in-line skating you must support your entire body weight. This constant load on the legs assists in developing your leg muscles specifically for this activity. During running, although your legs support your entire body weight, each time your foot contacts the ground it is subjected to forces equal to anywhere from two to six times your body weight—"pounding the pavement"; during in-line skating you "glide" repetitively, reducing joint stresses. This is clearly an advantage for individuals looking for an activity from which they can recover easily. For these and many other reasons, many people choose in-line skating

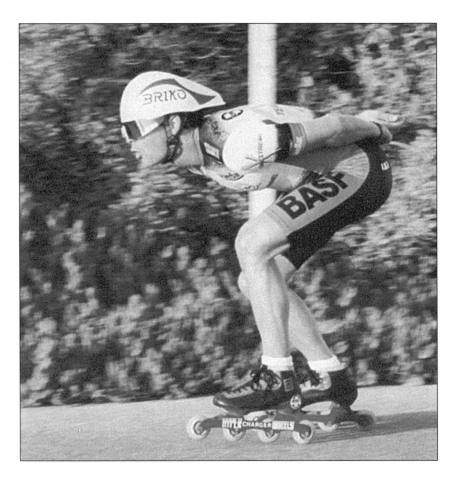

as a method of cross-training; it is a physically demanding yet enjoyable activity.

Research has demonstrated that in-line skating provides cardio-respiratory (heart rate and oxygen consumption) responses similar to those for other activities such as running and cycling. Effectively, that means you can use in-line skating to help you develop your cardiovascular fitness level. Many of the training programs used in other types of activities will work equally well with in-line skating; however, a few minor issues need to be addressed in order for you to optimize your workouts on skates.

Before You Start

In order to maximize your workouts, you'll need to determine a few things: your goals, equipment needs, and type of training. We'll consider your goals first since they will dictate both the equipment you will need and the type and intensity of your training.

Your Goals

Whether you choose to use in-line skating as a method of acquiring or maintaining fitness, or decide to actually enter in-line skate races, you'll need endurance; so a major focus of training will be on providing you with that endurance. If you'll be racing on in-line skates, you should additionally devote at least one session per week of training to speed workouts. If you'll be skating for general fitness or using skating for cross-training, you can skip speed workouts on skates and spend more time training with the sport in which you'll be participating or competing.

Equipment

You'll want to select skates that will meet your needs, whatever your goal. Your first and main concern in selecting skates should be comfort. Finding a boot that fits you comfortably while providing adequate ankle support is critical. Your foot should fit snugly in the boot; you should not be able to move your foot around in the boot, yet it should not be tight enough to cause discomfort. If the boot fits too loosely, you may get blisters or chafing of the skin; if it is too tight, you may experience foot cramps or lower-leg fatigue.

One of the major differences between boots designed for fitness and those designed for racing is the height of the cuff of the boot. A number of "fitness skates" are available that incorporate a midankle-height cuff, which is somewhat lower than that of conventional recreational skates but not quite as low as that of racing skates. A shorter cuff does not necessarily make a skate more comfortable, but it may allow unrestricted range of motion of your ankle as you bend down to skate faster. Make sure you try on a boot before purchasing; take it for a test-skate if possible. If you'll also be using your in-line skates for racing, you should really consider a boot with a lower-cut cuff; since you'll be in a crouched position while racing, you'll want the added flexibility.

As already noted, frame length is an important characteristic of in-line skates in terms of performance. Note that unless you'll be racing, you do *not* need five wheels on each frame. Four wheels is sufficient; however, for optimum performance, you will want to select four-wheel skates with longer-than-normal frames. Longer frames do not offer the responsiveness of a shorter frame, but they provide faster, smoother skating. If you're physically fit, you'll be skating faster than most recreational skaters, so you will need longer frames for both the stability at higher skating speeds and the longer strides that you will be taking in your higher-speed, higher-intensity workouts. The easiest way to determine whether a skate has an extended frame is to compare it to recreational skates; look at the distance between the wheels. You should notice at least a 1/2-inch space between the wheels; if the wheels are closer together than 1/2 inch, consider a longer frame. Typically, four-wheel extended frames are at least 10.5 inches in length; five-wheel frames are at least 12.5 inches in length (measured from front axle to rear axle).

Wheels are also very important; wheels that are 76–80 millimeters in diameter are a good choice for most fitness skaters. Smaller (72-millimeter) wheels tend to be good for maneuverability, especially in actions such as jumping over garbage cans, doing 360-degree spins, and making quick direction changes; but since you're interested in fitness, you'd be better off with a larger-diameter wheel. Larger wheels tend to roll faster and longer, provide a more comfortable ride, and last longer before they need to be replaced. Since you'll be using your in-line skates for fitness, you'll probably be putting more miles on your skates in an average month than most recreational skaters will in an entire year, so the extended life of the larger-diameter wheels should be an advantage.

Durometer (hardness rating of a wheel, noted by the letter *A* after the number) is also an important wheel characteristic. Most skaters will use a wheel with a durometer rating of 78A–82A for outdoor skating. Wheels with higher durometer ratings have harder urethane, and while they roll easier and don't wear out as fast, they offer less grip and shock-absorbing capacity than lower-durometer wheels. Heavier skaters should select higher-durometer wheels, since body weight affects the performance of wheels (a 78A wheel will feel softer for a 180-pound skater than it does for a 140-pound skater).

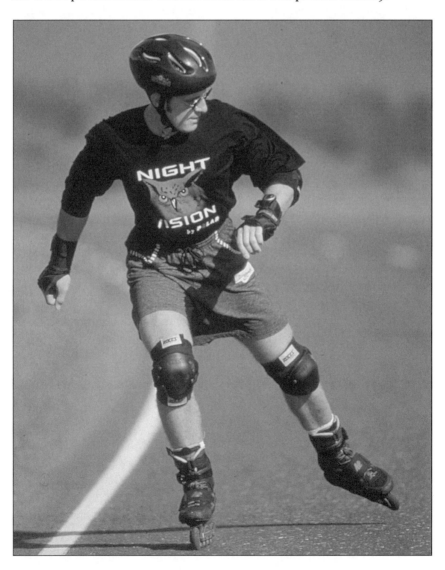

In terms of bearings, select a bearing that has an ABEC rating (ABEC is a group that sets worldwide standards for precision-bearing manufacture and tolerance). For in-line skate bearings, ABEC ratings are typically 1, 3, 5, and 7; the higher the ABEC rating, the higher the precision, as well as the price. Many skaters recommend the use of higher ABEC-rated bearings, but any quality ABEC-rated bearing is typically suitable for fitness in-line skating, and the increased cost of higher ABEC-rated bearings may not be justified in relation to increased performance.

Of course, the most important equipment for any in-line skater is protective gear, including a helmet, wrist guards, and knee and elbow pads.

Using Heart Rate Monitoring for In-Line Skating

In most activities, an increase in workload leads to an increase in oxygen consumption level (calorie burning), which is associated with an increase in heart rate. This heart rate-oxygen consumption relationship (relative heart rate) applies to in-line skating as well; however, under certain conditions the relationship may be somewhat skewed. During in-line skating under these conditions, your oxygen consumption level may be lower at any given heart rate than it is for other activities. This means that in order to achieve the same cardiovascular training effect during in-line skating, you may need to maintain your heart rate at a somewhat elevated level. It appears that the relative heart rate response may be affected by a number of factors, including the following.

- **Skating surface.** Softer surface = higher relative heart rate.
- **Frame length.** Longer frames = higher or lower relative heart rate depending on the speed of the skating.
- **Body position.** Bent-over body position = higher or lower relative heart rate. (This may be related to both the restriction of blood flow that is associated with the bent-knee position and the static nature of the glide phase of the stroke, especially in faster skaters, who may spend more time in the static phase of the stroke.)

The factors of frame length and body position may be related: skaters who have longer frames can more comfortably skate in the bent-over position, in part because of the stability of the longer frames.

Associated with the frame length and body position is another unique response of heart rate to in-line skating. When you are skating at a *slow to moderate pace* in the bent-over position, your heart rate and oxygen consumption may both be *higher* than when you skate upright at the same speed. At first glance, this appears strange, because at *higher* speeds your heart rate and oxygen consumption levels are both typically *lower* if you adopt the bent-over position. In large part the reason for the lower heart rate in this case is that during skating in the bent-over position your body is in a more aerodynamic position, reducing your wind resistance; at higher speeds, this means that less work needs to be done to keep you moving forward. At lower speeds, aerodynamics don't have a significant effect on energy cost (oxygen consumption); so the bent-over position is not effective in reducing the energy cost of skating, while the restricted blood flow to the legs that accompanies the bent-over position increases the heart rate.

Absolute heart rate (heart rate irrespective of oxygen consumption cost) is also influenced during skating by obvious factors such as your skating speed, the grade on which you skate (uphill = higher absolute heart rate), and other factors (table 6.1). Remember that while your absolute heart rate increases, you cannot be certain of the effect on oxygen consumption; and under certain conditions, the difference can be fairly large. But for most conditions, you can get a fairly accurate idea of the calorie-burning costs associated with various skating speeds (fig. 6.1). It is clear that oxygen consumption increases as skating speed increases, but for competitive skaters the oxygen consumption level for any speed is lower. This is probably due to a variety of factors, including characteristics associated with "competitive" skaters: longer frames, bent-over body position, and the use of larger, harder wheels, and drafting.

If you are accustomed to training at a particular heart rate, you might find that by using the same heart rate during in-line skating you feel as though you're not working as hard. This may occur if you're skating on a soft surface, using long frames, or skating in the bent position at higher skating speeds. Simply bump up your heart rate a few beats to adjust for the different heart rate response.

TABLE 6.1	Factors That Influence Absolute Heart Rate

Variable	Effect on HR
Drafting	↓
Soft skating surface	↑
Longer frames	↑ ↓
Bent-over position	↑ ↓
Larger wheel diameter	↓
Harder wheels	↓
Higher speed	↑
Higher body weight	↑
Carrying load (backpack, etc.)	↑
Skating uphill	↑

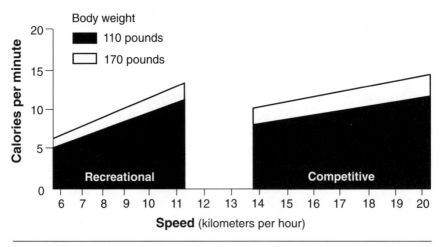

Figure 6.1 Calories burned per minute during in-line skating.

Finding Your Optimal Training Intensity for Skating

In-line skating elicits a unique set of physical perceptions: Your legs get tired because of the unusual semi-static position during the glide phase of your stride, your lower back becomes fatigued from being bent over, and your neck muscles sometimes become tired since you need to keep your head up in order to see where you're skating. All of this activity can produce a set of perceptions very different from that for other sports you may be more familiar with.

The rating of perceived exertion (RPE) is somewhat useful for most activities—but to a limited extent. With the RPE you simply rate your level of effort at any given time during an activity and use it to guide your exercise. If you feel that you're working "very easy," you may need to pick up the pace; if you think the exercise is "very hard," you might choose to decrease your intensity. While the RPE method of determining your intensity doesn't require any equipment, it also does not take into account the myriad factors that may have an effect on your perception of effort. Since in-line skating can induce a number of unusual sensations as described earlier, a more objective measurement of intensity, or body effort, is helpful. That measurement, of course, is the heart rate.

Before you set a heart rate range for your training regimen, you need to know your maximal heart rate (MHR). As described in chapters 1 and 2, your MHR is the fastest that your heart can beat normally. To determine your actual MHR, you can use one of the prediction formulas provided, or, in the case of in-line skating, you can take an increasing skating-pace test. If you want to determine your MHR while skating, you have two options: (1) take the "hill-climb test" if you have access to a long hill or (2) take the "sprint test," using a long, straight stretch of road.

Hill-Climb Test

For this test, you'll need to find a hill that you cannot climb in less than 4 minutes. Warm up by skating on a relatively flat road for 5–10 minutes at a moderate pace. Then, beginning at the bottom of a long hill, begin your ascent, increasing your pace so that you achieve your maximum sustainable uphill speed within the first 2 minutes, while checking your heart rate monitor. Increase your pace to almost a sprint for another minute or so, glancing at your monitor every few seconds to note the heart rate. Finally, sprint for 30 seconds to 1 minute and note the highest heart rate you achieve.

Highest heart rate = _____ (MHR)

Sprint Test

If you don't live in a hilly area, you can perform another test that is similar to the hill-climb test. First, you need to make sure you have plenty of traffic-free space in which to do this test; you'll be quite tired and probably won't be paying attention to cars. Begin by performing a warm-up similar to that for the hill-climb test. When you're adequately warmed up, gradually increase your pace for two minutes until you reach your maximum sustainable speed. Next, start to skate faster, swinging your arms to increase your speed to a near-sprint pace for at least two minutes, while occasionally looking at your heart rate monitor. Make a final sprint of 30 seconds to one minute, pumping your arms to help you skate as fast as possible. Note your MHR.

Highest heart rate = _____ (MHR)

Now that you have your MHR, you are almost ready to set up your training heart rate ranges. You need one other piece of information—your resting heart rate (RHR). Take your RHR on five consecutive mornings before getting out of bed. Simply use your heart rate monitor, and while lying in bed, note your RHR. The

average of five consecutive mornings will give you a good represen-
tation of your RHR.

Resting heart rate = _____ (RHR)

To determine your training heart rate ranges, perform the following calculations:
Determine your heart rate reserve (HRR):

MHR – RHR

_____ = HRR

Using this information, perform the following calculations:

Easy Training Heart Rate Range (zone 1)
(HRR × .55) + RHR   –   (HRR × .6) + RHR

_____   –   _____

Aerobic Training Heart Rate Range (zone 2)
(HRR × .61) + RHR   –   (HRR × .7) + RHR

_____   –   _____

Steady State Training Heart Rate Range (zone 3)
(HRR × .71) + RHR   –   (HRR × .8) + RHR

_____   –   _____

Anaerobic Threshold Training Heart Rate Range (zone 4)
(HRR × .81) + RHR   –   (HRR × .9) + RHR

_____   –   _____

Competitive Training Heart Rate Range (zone 5)
(HRR × .91) + RHR   –   MHR

_____   –   _____

Keep in mind that with all of these workout ranges (except the
Competitive Training Heart Rate Range), you may need to keep
your heart rate a few beats *above* the numbers you've calculated
in order to maximize your cardiovascular fitness benefits. This is
true particularly if you skate on a soft surface, with longer frames,
or in the bent position as explained earlier.

Designing Your In-Line Skating Program

Easy Training Heart Rate Range workouts are designed to provide you with a relaxing, recovery-type exercise session while still improving fitness. You can use these workouts on days when you are recovering from a harder workout, or if you're just getting back into skating. Be very attentive to your heart rate during these workouts; it's easy to pick up speed and elevate your heart rate into the next training range; if this happens, slow down.

The next level, your Aerobic Training Heart Rate Range, is where you should spend most of your time in training. Although the intensity of these workouts is lower than in Steady State, Anaerobic Threshold, and Competitive Training Heart Rate Range workouts, they are still able to fulfill even the most demanding athlete's quest for "overall workout value" by being longer in duration. These workouts are light enough that you can do them and still concentrate on technique. When performing workouts that include the Aerobic Training Heart Rate Range, check your heart rate monitor

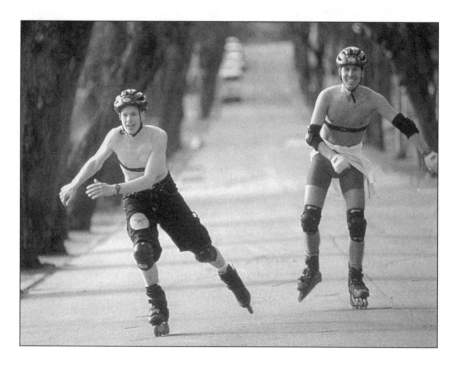

to make sure your heart rate is where it's supposed to be; it's easy to get carried away.

Steady State Training Heart Rate Range workouts make you feel as though you're getting a good workout; you'll be breathing heavier than in the Aerobic and Easy Training Heart Rate Range workouts and will experience some muscle fatigue, but these workouts are a necessity for improving your ability to hold a fast pace while skating. They require concentration on technique and maintenance of a consistent pace. If your heart rate goes higher than Steady State Training Heart Rate Range, you'll need to reduce your pace to optimize your benefits.

Anaerobic Threshold Training Heart Rate Range workouts focus more on pushing your limit of speed—they're difficult. When you engage in workouts and your heart rate reaches this range, you should skate only until you notice fatigue building in your muscles; allowing your legs to become too fatigued can lead to accidents (i.e., crossing your skates over each other and falling).

Finally, Competitive Training Heart Rate Range workouts are designed for those individuals who want to challenge themselves or for those who will be entering in-line skating races. Workouts that push your heart rate to the Competitive Training Heart Rate Range make you work beyond your anaerobic threshold; they are designed to develop strength and power. Therefore, they are not done for extended periods of time (you cannot effectively work at a pace above anaerobic threshold for very long).

Warm-Up

Warming up before any type of workout has a number of benefits. Since the demand for oxygenated blood in exercising muscles is increased with physical activity, the blood vessels supplying those muscles require a few minutes to dilate in order to facilitate this increased blood flow. In addition, because of the unique nature of the movements while in-line skating, you may find that warming up before skating is particularly beneficial. During in-line skating the range of motion of your legs can change dramatically, unlike what happens in other sports such as cycling, where the range of motion remains fairly consistent irrespective of the intensity of the activity. Shorter strides, longer strides, sitting "deeper," pushing longer, and making quick direction changes are all common during in-line skating. Because of the physiologic demands and unique movement patterns associated with in-line skating, inadequate warm-up can increase your risk of muscular injury.

A good warm-up for in-line skating is to skate slowly for 5–10 minutes at a pace that will increase your heart rate to your Easy Training Heart Rate Range (55–60 percent). During this time, your breathing will become somewhat deeper and faster, and your body will respond to the effort further by increasing blood flow to both your lower back muscles and your leg muscles. This warm-up helps prepare your body for the workout that will follow.

Cool-Down

Cooling down is an important part of any workout; in-line skating is no exception. During the cool-down period, the blood flow to the working muscles is decreased gradually as the demand for oxygenated blood is reduced. This in turn leads to a constriction of the blood vessels in the working muscles to a more normal resting

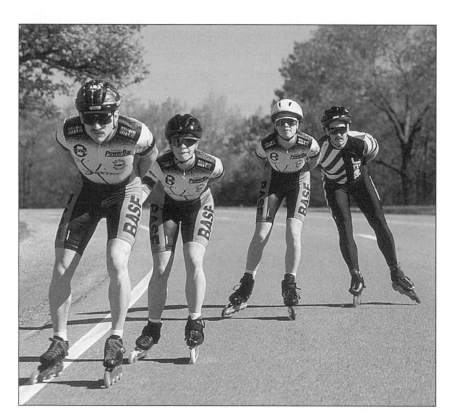

diameter. These blood vessel changes require a few minutes, so cooling down is an important part of any well-designed workout regimen.

An adequate cool-down after an in-line skating workout usually consists of skating for 5–10 minutes at a pace that allows your heart rate to come back down to your Easy Training Heart Rate Range (55–60 percent), or to within about 20–30 beats above your preexercise heart rate.

Adjusting Intensity in Your Skating Workouts

Before any workout, make sure you're wearing your protective gear. Next, check to make sure your skates are in good working condition: check your wheels and bearings, brakes, and laces and buckles. Finally, put on your heart rate monitor and get ready to work out!

When used properly, the following five workouts form the basis for a complete fitness in-line skating training program. Endurance, speed, power, and pacing are all addressed; and the training program follows a hard/easy schedule (you don't do hard workouts on two consecutive days). Even with the more intense workouts included, for some skaters the duration of the workouts listed will not provide a sufficient challenge. If that happens for you, simply increase the duration of the workouts (except for workouts 2 and 5) to meet your requirements, but don't increase the intensity; each workout has specific goals in terms of intensity. Table 6.2 gives a key to the heart rate ranges used in the workouts.

Keep in mind that all of your workouts do not need to be as structured as these plans. You can use these workouts as a guide, and once you've achieved a reasonable level of fitness, can modify your schedule to keep your program fun. Remember, in-line skating should be an enjoyable activity, not something that is regimented and rigid.

Workout 1—Endurance

Workout: 30 minutes in zone 2. Warm up and cool down as needed.

This workout is designed to help you improve your endurance while skating at a pace sufficient to help you develop leg strength.

TABLE 6.2	Key to Heart Rate Ranges	
Zone	Description	Percent MHR
	Warm-up/cool-down level	50–60 (or 20–30 beats above rest)
Zone 1	Easy training heart rate range	55–60
Zone 2	Aerobic training heart rate range	61–70
Zone 3	Steady state training heart rate range	71–80
Zone 4	Anaerobic threshold training heart rate range	81–90
Zone 5	Competitive training heart rate range	91–100

The duration of your longest endurance workout should be increased by 10 minutes every two weeks for the first six weeks, then by 20 minutes every two weeks until you reach a total time of 120 minutes. If you find that you're having a difficult time getting skating at a pace that allows your heart rate to reach this range without working hard, you are not ready to increase the duration of the workout; you need to continue at the duration you've reached until skating in this range doesn't cause undue fatigue.

Workout 2—Recovery

Workout: 40 minutes in zone 1. Warm up and cool down as needed.

This is a workout you can use at any time during your training, especially when you feel that you may be "overdoing it" a bit and need to take a day to skate easy. Watch your heart rate during the entire workout; if you're maintaining the same pace and you notice that your heart rate is climbing, consider skating with a more upright body position and slowing down. Many athletes don't think that they are working hard enough to benefit from this type of workout. Don't worry—you'll be skating long enough to burn a reasonable number of calories, while at the same time skating at a level of intensity sufficient to help you maintain and possibly even improve your fitness level. The duration of this workout should be increased only to a maximum of 45 minutes. The goal of this workout is to help with recovery, and exercising for an extended duration won't allow you to completely recover. Take particular note of your recovery heart rate within about 5 minutes of your cool-down. It should come back down quite fast; if not, you may be overdoing it with your training schedule and may need to either repeat this workout on your next scheduled workout day or schedule a day of complete rest.

Workout 3—Speed

Workout: 3 minutes in zone 4 followed by 6 minutes in zone 3; repeat for a total workout time of 40–60 minutes. Warm up and cool down as needed.

This workout will help you learn to skate faster for an increasingly longer period of time. The format—skating for 3 minutes with your heart rate in your Anaerobic Threshold Training Heart Rate Range, followed by 6 minutes of skating with your heart rate in your Steady State Training Heart Rate Range—can be gradually extended to make a workout of up to 60 minutes in duration. This should not be done until you have been following a training program for at least four to six weeks. As your fitness level improves, your pace during each of these segments will increase. The 3-minute segments will provide you with enough intensity to tire you out, followed by the 6-minute segment that will allow you to recover enough for your next 3-minute Anaerobic Threshold segment.

TRAINING PLAN

FITNESS WORKOUT PROGRAM
(FIRST TWO-WEEK CYCLE)

S	M	T	W	Th	F	S	
1	3	2	R	1	2	R	3 hours
2	3	1	2	R	3	1	3 hours, 40 minutes

Notes: R = rest day
The workouts listed should be done for the durations indicated; do not do extended versions of these workouts for the first two-week cycle unless you have been skating for more than four hours per week already.

Workout 4—Speed Play

Workout: 30 minutes in zone 2 with occasional sprints in zone 5. Warm up and cool down as needed.

During this workout, you can use your heart rate monitor as a timer, and have a friend skate with you and perform two or three "sprints" away from you over the course of a 30-minute workout. The goal is to make a game of skating fast during your workout. You should strive to maintain a heart rate in your Aerobic Training Heart Rate Range during the majority of the workout, with interspersed bursts of high-intensity skating. Regardless of whether or not you're skating with a partner, make sure your heart rate reaches the Competitive Training Heart Rate Range during each burst, striving to hold that pace for approximately 1 minute. Then, reduce your speed until your heart rate reaches your Aerobic Training Heart Rate Range, and maintain that pace for at least 8–10 minutes before another burst of speed. This workout can be extended to 60 minutes in duration as your fitness level improves.

Workout 5—Time Trial

Workout: 30 minutes in zone 4. Warm up and cool down as needed.

The goal of this workout is to push yourself to perform at the highest level you can for a 30-minute period—similar to what you would do in a 10K in-line skate race. Most competitive fitness skaters finish a 10K in 30 minutes or less, so if you perform this workout regularly, you should have no problem completing a 10K. Do this workout at least once every three to four weeks, as often as once every two weeks if you plan on competing. It teaches you to skate at or near your anaerobic threshold. Using your heart rate monitor as the determinant of your pace, keep your heart rate in your Anaerobic Threshold Training Heart Rate Range for the entire 30 minutes. Consistency is key; don't go too fast during the start of the workout or you will have difficulty completing the 30 minutes without slowing down excessively.

FITNESS WORKOUT PROGRAM
(SECOND TWO-WEEK CYCLE)

S	M	T	W	Th	F	S	TOTAL
R	4	2	1e	2	R	5	3 hours
2	3	R	4e	1e	2	1	3 hours, 50 minutes

Notes: R = rest day
e = extended duration (increase by 10 minutes over previous two-week cycle).

FITNESS WORKOUT PROGRAM
(THIRD TWO-WEEK CYCLE)

S	M	T	W	Th	F	S	TOTAL
2+	R	3e	2	1	4e	2	4 hours, 15 minutes
R	3e	1e	2	3e	R	4e	4 hours

Notes: R = rest day
e = extended duration (increase by 10 minutes over previous two-week cycle).
2+ = workout 2, 45-minute duration.

FITNESS WORKOUT PROGRAM
(FOURTH TWO-WEEK CYCLE)

S	M	T	W	Th	F	S	TOTAL
3e	R	5	2+	1e	2+	3e	4 hours, 40 minutes
R	3e	2+	4e	R	3e	1e	4 hours, 15 minutes

Notes: R = rest day
e = extended duration (increase by 10 minutes over previous two-week cycle).
2+ = workout 2, 45-minute duration.

Although the workouts I have described do not cover all of the possible conditions in which you'll skate, you can modify them to suit your situation. For example, if you live in an area with lots of hills, substitute hill climbs in workouts 3 and 4. To get more adept at skating with a partner, do some drafting drills by skating directly behind someone. To improve your technique, practice gliding longer and lengthening your strides. Have some fun in your workouts. But more important than the type of workouts you do, you need to make sure you do them consistently and with respect for your body's ability to recover. Remember that recovery is a key component to any well-rounded fitness program, so make sure you incorporate recovery sessions and rest days into your training program.

If you will listen to your body's responses to exercise (paying particular attention to your heart rate, breathing rate, recovery heart rate, and muscle fatigue), you can make great strides in improving or maintaining your fitness level. If you follow the basic guidelines outlined in this chapter, you will be well on your way to a rewarding experience— a lifetime of fitness in-line skating! Stay healthy and happy.

CHAPTER 7

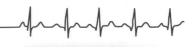

MULTISPORT TRAINING

TIMOTHY J. MOORE

Anyone seeking an athletic challenge need look no further than multisport competition. What started out as fringe events among fitness fanatics has grown into organized competitions such as triathlons (swim, bike, run) and duathlons (run, bike, run). Not to be outdone, winter sport enthusiasts have devised contests that include some of their favorite disciplines (cross-country skiing, snowshoeing, and skating). Outdoor adventurers have assembled demanding tests of mind and body that include paddling, mountain biking, rock climbing and mountaineering, and horseback riding, among others.

Getting the Most From Your Multisport Program

A properly designed training program has many functions, including improving your performance, preventing burnout, and reducing the risk of injuries. Therefore it is very important that you understand the various principles that go into the design and implementation of your training routine.

The Laws of Training

There are some basic rules of training that you will need to understand if you want to get the most from your multisport program. The first is called the *law of overload*. Simply put, if your goal is to get into better competitive shape, you need to continually increase the quantity and quality of your workouts. The law states that when an individual is exposed to stress (called a "load"), fatigue is produced. When the loading stops, a recovery process follows in which the individual "supercompensates" to a higher level of fitness as shown in figure 7.1. Thus, increases in training loads cause the body to adapt to the stress placed upon it by getting stronger. But you must properly alternate your training loads in order to achieve optimum results.

The next concept that you will need to grasp is the *law of reversibility*. Here the basic idea is the concept of "move it or lose it." So, if you do not work out at a high enough intensity, you will not be performing at your best in races. You must continually challenge yourself by changing your training load as your fitness level improves—a rule also known as the "principle of increasing demands."

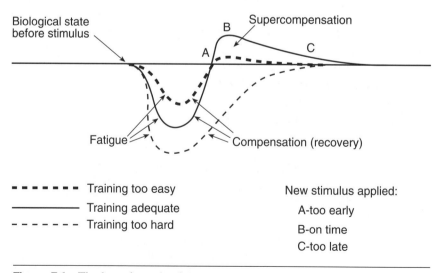

Figure 7.1   The law of overload.

The final rule for you to learn is the *law of specificity.* This just means that if you plan on competing in an open-water swim, for example, you should not do all your training in a swimming pool. In addition, to be successful you have to train the energy system, or the different energy systems, used in the activities that you will be competing in, so it's good to be as specialized as possible with your training. This is called the SAID principle, or "specific adaptation to imposed demands."

Periodization

In addition to the laws of training, one of the biggest lessons for someone who works out regularly to learn is that rest is just as important as exercise. Developing a system that helps regulate the amount of stress we place on our bodies through exercise, with properly placed rest periods, is the key to a successful training program. For years, eastern European athletes have dominated amateur sport competitions such as the Olympics using a technique known as periodization. It consists of a planned system of alternating the intensity (quality) and volume (quantity) of your workouts throughout the year to achieve optimum results, as in the schedule shown in figure 7.2.

Intensity or effort is the strength of a training load, or concentration of work per unit of time (quality). You can gauge your intensity by using your heart rate to monitor your cardiovascular workouts, as well as keeping track of the amount of weight you lift during strength-training sessions.

Volume or duration is the extent or amount (quantity) of training performed during a particular workout. It can be determined by the

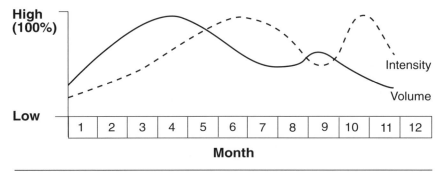

Figure 7.2 Structure of a periodized year, showing alternating volume and intensity.

number of miles or minutes you cover each week in your cardiovascular workouts, or the total number of minutes you put in at the gym lifting weights every week. It is important to remember that these two variables are inversely proportional to each other. For example, if your volume is high, it is difficult to also maintain a high level of intensity, and vice versa.

Training Terminology

The basic building blocks of the systematic approach of periodization include the following important terms:

A *training session* is a typical training day in your workout schedule. It consists of (1) warm-up and flexibility, (2) energy-system work (either aerobic or anaerobic), (3) neuromuscular work (such as strength or skill/technique training), and (4) cool-down and flexibility.

A *microcycle* is a group of training sessions organized in such a way that they produce an optimal training effect. A microcycle generally lasts for a week, with a specific number of training sessions based on your fitness level, age, experience, and other factors such as time limitations. The microcycles are planned so that variations in the volume (quantity) and intensity (quality) of training occur throughout the year in an effort to prevent over-training; see the samples shown in figures 7.3 and 7.4.

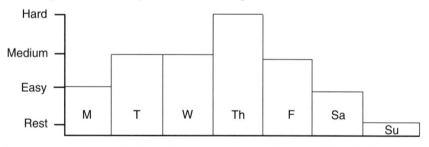

Figure 7.3 A week-long microcycle with one peak.

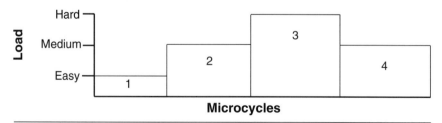

Figure 7.4 A group of macrocycles, showing the increase of training load in steps.

Proper recovery must be allowed by including lower-intensity days such as "active-rest" workouts like easy swimming or cycling. This is critical to your performance, since a recent study showed that low-intensity activity consisting of easy cycling demonstrated 50 percent less lactic acid (an unwanted by-product of exercise that causes stiffness) buildup than was seen in those individuals who just rested.

Designing Your Multisport Program

When you are designing the cardiovascular portion of your training program, you should use the principles of periodization to alternate the volume and intensity of your workouts. For example, you can change the intensity or effort of your training sessions by alternating the percentage of your heart rate at which you are exercising:

Monday: hard (85 percent of maximal heart rate)

Wednesday: easy (65 percent of maximal heart rate)

Friday: medium (75 percent of maximal heart rate)

Thus you can perform an interval session at over 80 percent of your maximal heart rate on one day, a recovery or active-rest workout at around 60 percent on another, and a distance or endurance workout at between 70 to 80 percent of your maximal heart rate on a third day.

In addition, you can alter the volume of your training sessions by varying the duration or total time of your workouts, with longer efforts generally representing more stressful days:

Monday: hard (2-hour-long ride)

Wednesday: easy (20-minute swim)

Friday: medium (45-minute run)

Finally, you can also vary the types of activities you are doing, since some forms of aerobic exercise are more stressful than others. For example, running involves higher-impact forces and therefore can be more stressful than cycling, while swimming may be easier on the body than riding your bike:

Monday: hard (run)

Wednesday: easy (swim)

Friday: medium (bike)

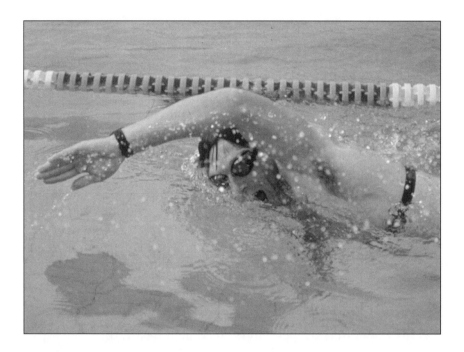

When developing a comprehensive training program, an athlete should always break up the year into off-season, preseason, in-season, and transition phases.

Off-Season Training

During the off-season, general overall training is carried out. Sometime this phase is referred to as "training to train." It lays the foundation for the harder training that will follow. This period consists mostly of continuous, increasingly longer efforts performed at 60 to 75 percent of an individual's maximal heart rate. The effects of training on the body at this time include increased carbohydrate reserves in the liver and muscle, better oxygen-carrying capacity, and the ability to burn fat more efficiently.

Also during this phase, you should include other forms of cardiovascular exercise such as mountain biking and in-line skating, since they help train your agility, balance, and coordination (skill training) for better all-around performance. The one important rule to follow during this, or any other phase, is never to raise your total mileage more than 10 percent from week to week; this will help you avoid injury from rapid increases in volume.

Preseason Training

This is the toughest time for training, since it involves combining some of the higher-mileage training from the off-season with more race pace-type workout sessions. During the preseason phase, training consists mainly of higher-intensity aerobic workouts (a mix of both aerobic and anaerobic energy development) that concentrate on the specific energy systems that will be used during an actual multisport competition. Interval training is used to improve both your maximal oxygen consumption ($\dot{V}O_2$max) and lactate threshold (LT), with the longer $\dot{V}O_2$ workouts receiving priority during the beginning of the phase. As an example, a $\dot{V}O_2$ workout could involve efforts at over 85 percent of your maximal heart rate for around 8 to 10 minutes, with short rest periods of several minutes.

Lactate threshold work, on the other hand, usually lasts from five to eight minutes, at around 80 percent (or above) of your maximal heart rate, with equal periods of active rest (easy jogging or cycling) to help with the removal of lactic acid. Because of genetic limitations there is a ceiling to the increases that can be produced through $\dot{V}O_2$ training, but the good news is that your LT can be affected to a much greater degree. This is an important point, since your LT has been shown to be a good predictor of endurance performance in sports like the triathlon. That's because a higher LT allows you work at a faster pace over longer periods of time.

One important thing you can do to improve your performance during hard training is to put two higher-intensity workouts back-to-back while including at least two days of rest between your harder days. That's because research has shown that following such a schedule can help increase the blood volume in your body, an important factor for endurance performance. The first hard workout causes this effect by increasing the volume of blood in your body, which then allows you to have a better workout on the second hard session.

In addition, including two days of rest between higher-intensity training sessions prevents you from having to work out on the exact day that your muscle soreness peaks. Remember, delayed-onset muscle soreness is worse 48 hours after a workout, so if you used a hard/easy training format, you would be doing your next hard session just in time to have to deal with completing a workout when you are stiff and sore. Lastly, during this phase, for some added variety you can substitute running and cycling on hilly courses in place of your harder interval-training sessions. Also, don't forget your warm-ups and cool-downs.

In-Season Training

Finally, to bring you to a "peak," your interval work must be done at a pace slightly quicker than what you would be doing during the

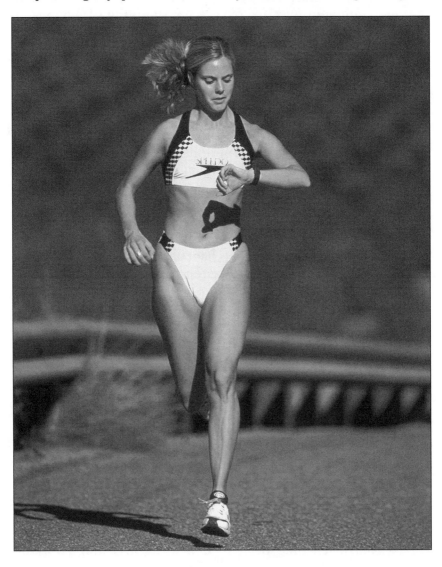

race. This means that your interval sessions will become shorter, faster, and harder (90 percent of your maximal heart rate and above). Also during this time, it is important to reduce the number of miles or yards that you are doing per week, to help with the peaking process and prevent burnout.

In addition, during this phase many triathletes perform what are known as "brick" workouts that simulate the bike-to-run transition. A brick usually consists of at least an 8- to 10-mile ride immediately followed by a 2- to 3-mile run, but both of these can be shorter. This type of training helps save some wear and tear on your legs, since you don't have to run as far to get a good workout. That's because you are already fatigued from riding the bike.

You can also link up other events such as swimming and cycling by using an upper-body ergometer followed by a stationary cycle. This helps train the multisport athlete for the transition from upper-body to lower-body exercise. This is an important point, since fatigue in the legs occurs earlier if previous exercise with the arms has raised the level of lactic acid circulating in the blood (especially for athletes with more fast-twitch fibers). One final tip to follow during this phase is that rest is almost as important as training, maybe more so. So allow enough recovery time after your hard workouts to achieve your best performances.

Transition Phase

The last part of the program consists of about a month of low-intensity activities (below 75 percent of your maximal heart rate). The goal is to physically and mentally recover from a long year of training. The best thing you can do during this time to ensure meeting that goal is to pick an activity that you did not do during the year and do it—such as taking a hike in the woods, doing a little paddling down a quiet river in the wilderness, or even playing an easy set of tennis. Also, don't forget your mental recovery; go out and buy that murder mystery you have been wanting to read, listen to some music, or take a weekend getaway. Choose activities that you find relaxing and enjoyable.

Adjusting Intensity in Your Multisport Program

No matter what phase of training you are in, it is important to vary the intensity of your workouts during any given week. A typical program will include a harder day of working out such as interval training, a recovery (rest) or easy day, and a medium-intensity or endurance workout cycled throughout the week. When performing any high-intensity work such as your interval training, always include a good warm-up and cool-down that incorporate a little stretching to help reduce delayed-onset muscle soreness.

Also, if you find that you are not able to perform your prescribed workout on any given day, adjust your schedule accordingly by either skipping the workout or doing an easy session instead. Learning to make such changes will not only give you a better understanding of your training and your body, but will also result in improved performances and a reduced risk of injury.

Sample Training Program

Here is an 18-week training program that I have designed to help prepare you for an Olympic-distance triathlon; the same training principles, though, can be used in other multisport events. Training heart rate intensities in this program follow the four-zone system laid out by Dr. Burke in chapter 2, using the maximal heart rate and LT tests discussed in the running and cycling chapters to help determine your percentages. To figure out your maximal heart rate in swimming, perform an all-out 200-yard effort after a good warm-up of 10 minutes. Your heart rate at the end of the sprint is your maximum, although individuals who are more fit might require a slightly longer distance to get their heart rate up to their max.

TRAINING PLAN

OFF-SEASON
(BASE PHASE)

Eight weeks

MONDAY

A.M.- *Weight training*; free weights (hard).

P.M.- *Bike*; medium ride of 60 to 90 minutes at 65 to 75 of your maximum.

TUESDAY

A.M.- *Run*; medium run of 30 to 45 minutes at 65 to 75 percent of your maximum.

P.M.- *Swim*; long swim of 35 to 50 minutes at 60 to 70 percent of your maximum.

WEDNESDAY

A.M.- *Weight training*; machines (easy).

P.M.- *Bike*; long ride of 90 to 120 minutes at 65 to 75 percent of your maximum.

THURSDAY

A.M.- *Run*; medium run of 30 to 45 minutes at 65 to 75 percent of your maximum.

P.M.- *Swim*; drills: Warm up 400 yards; main set of two times 50 yards of kicking on stomach, two times 50 yards kicking on back, two times 50 yards kicking on side (both sides), two times 50 yards one-arm drill (both sides), two times 50 yards catch-up drill. Sprint set of six to eight times 25 yards (concentrate on good form, no heart rate) with a one-to-two work:rest ratio. Recovery heart rate below 65 percent of your maximum on sprints. Cool down 200 yards.

FRIDAY

A.M.- *Weight training*; free weights (medium).

P.M.- *Bike*; medium ride of 60 to 90 minutes at 65 to 75 percent of your maximum.

SATURDAY

Rest.

SUNDAY

A.M.-*Run*; long run of 45 to 60 minutes at 65 to 75 percent of your maximum.

P.M.-*Swim*; long swim of 35 to 45 minutes at 60 to 70 percent of your maximum.

M	Tu	W	Th	F	Sa	Su
Weights	Run	Weights	Run	Weights	Rest	Run
(Hard)	(Med.)	(Easy)	(Med.)	(Med.)		(Dist.)
Bike	Swim	Bike	Swim	Bike		Swim
(Med.)	(Dist.)	(Dist.)	(Med.)	(Med.)		(Dist.)

TRAINING PLAN

PRESEASON
(STRENGTH PHASE)

Six weeks

MONDAY

A.M.- *Weight training*; free weights (hard).

P.M.-*Run*; long run of 45 to 60 minutes at 65 to 75 percent of your maximum.

TUESDAY

WEEKS 1-3

A.M.- *Swim;* easy recovery workout of 20 to 25 minutes of lap swimming with stroke and kick drills, heart rate at 60 to 70 percent of your maximum.

WEEKS 1-6

A.M.-*Bike;* hill training: Warm up 10 miles; two sets of two to four repeats, 8 to 12 percent grade, 200 to 400 meters in length; maintain 50–70 revolutions per minute. For first two repeats, use optimum gearing; try to stay seated. Third repeat should be done slightly overgeared, while for your last repeat you should stand up for the last half of the hill. All training heart rates should be at 80 to 90 percent of your maximum. Allow 5 minutes' rest between repeats, and 8 to 10 minutes between sets with easy spinning at a heart rate of below 120 beats per minute. Cool down 10 miles.

WEEKS 4–5

Bike; LT intervals: Warm up 10 miles; two to four times 3 miles, at 80 to 90 percent of your maximum. Rest two to four minutes, spinning in small chain ring (holding 65 percent of maximum for at least two minutes). Cool down 10 miles.

WEEK 6

Bike/Run; brick workout: Warm up five minutes on bike; then do a 15-mile bike ride immediately followed by 3-mile run, both at 80 to 90 percent of your maximum. Cool down 10 miles.

WEDNESDAY

WEEKS 1–3

A.M.- *Run;* hill training: Warm up one to two miles; six to eight times 200 yards on a steep hill (30 to 40 degrees) at a heart rate of 80 to 90 percent of your maximum at the end of each repeat. Jog-down recovery (one-to-four work:rest ratio, heart rate below 120). Cool down one to two miles.

WEEKS 4–6

A.M.- *Run;* "cruise intervals": Warm up one to two miles; two times 8 to 10 minutes at 80 to 90 percent of your maximum. Rest for 3 minutes by running an easy pace (heart rate below 120). Cool down one to two miles.

WEEKS 1–6

P.M.- *Bike;* medium ride of 60 to 90 minutes at 65 to 75 percent of your maximum.

THURSDAY

A.M.- *Weight training;* machines (easy).

P.M.- *Swim;* long swim of 35 to 45 minutes at 65 to 75 percent of your maximum.

FRIDAY

Rest.

SATURDAY

WEEKS 1–3

A.M.-*Run;* medium run of 30 to 45 minutes at 65 to 75 percent of your maximum.

WEEKS 1–6

P.M.-*Swim;* interval workout: Warm up 400 yards; main set of two to three times 400 yards at near race pace with a heart rate of 80 to 90 percent of your maximum, with three to five minutes' rest in between at a heart rate of below 65 percent of your maximum. Kick and stroke drills. Sprint set of three to five times 50 yards with a one-to-two work:rest ratio, recovery heart rate below 65 percent of your maximum. Cool down 200 yards.

WEEKS 4–6

Swim; interval workout: Warm up 400 yards; main set of 10 to 12 times 100 yards at 5 seconds slower than race pace at a heart rate of 75 to 85 percent of your maximum, with 10 to 15 seconds' rest in between at a heart rate below 65 percent of your maximum. Kick and stroke drills. Sprint set of 8 to 10 times 25 yards (all out; no heart rate) with a one-to-two work:rest ratio, heart rate below 65 percent of your maximum. Cool down 200 yards.

SUNDAY

Bike; long ride of 90 to 120 minutes at 65 to 75 percent of your maximum.

M	Tu	W	Th	F	Sa	Su
Weights	Swim	Run	Weights	Rest	Run	Bike
(Hard)	(Easy)	(Hard)	(Easy)		(Med.)	(Dist.)
Run	Bike	Bike	Swim		Swim	
(Dist.)	(Hard)	(Med.)	(Dist.)		(Hard)	

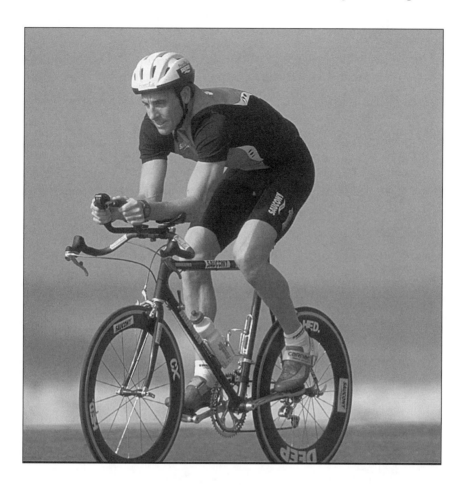

TRAINING PLAN

IN-SEASON
(SPEED)

Three weeks

MONDAY

Run; medium-intensity run of 30 to 45 minutes at 65 to 75 percent of your maximum.

TUESDAY

Swim; easy recovery workout of 20- to 25-minute lap swimming with stroke and kick drills at 60 to 70 percent of your maximum.

WEDNESDAY

WEEKS 1–2

Run; interval workout: Warm up one mile; three times one-mile repeats at 10 seconds faster than race pace at a heart rate of 85 to 95 percent of your maximum; 880-yard-jog recovery (heart rate below 65 percent of maximum). Cool down one mile.

WEEK 3

Run; interval workout: Warm up one mile; six times 880 yards at five seconds faster than race pace for a heart rate of 85 to 95 percent of your maximum; 440-yard-jog recovery (heart rate below 65 percent of maximum). Cool down one mile.

THURSDAY

Bike; medium of 45 to 60 minutes at 65 to 75 percent of your maximum.

FRIDAY

Rest.

SATURDAY

WEEKS 1–2

Swim; interval workout: Warm up 400 yards; main set of three sets of five times 50 yards with your heart rate at 85 to 95 percent of your maximum at end of repeat, with 60 seconds' rest between repeats (heart rate below 65 percent of your maximum), three to five minutes between sets. Kick and stroke drills. Cool down 200 yards.

WEEK 3

Swim; interval workout: Warm up 400 yards; main set of 10 times 25 yards with fins at faster than race pace (no heart rate). Rest for 60 to 90 seconds with your heart rate below 65 percent of your maximum. Kick and stroke drills. Cool down 200 yards.

SUNDAY

WEEK 1

Bike; declining sprints (anaerobic power): Warm up 10 miles; two times 60, 50, 40, 30, 20 seconds, done in your big chain ring at a heart rate of 85 to 95 percent of your maximum. Full recovery of two to four minutes (heart rate of below 65 percent of maximum) spinning in small chain ring. Cool down 10 miles.

WEEK 2

Bike; sprints (speed/anaerobic training): Warm up 10 miles; two sets of three to five repeats of 10 to 20 seconds all out (no heart rate). Complete rest of 5 minutes or more between repeats, and at least 10 minutes between sets at a heart rate of below 65 percent of maximum. Use a downhill grade during the last couple of training sessions. Cool down 10 miles.

WEEK 3

Bike/Run; brick workout: Warm up one mile running; then do 5 minutes on the bike ride on a wind trainer, immediately followed by a 440-yard run on the track. Repeat two to four times, keeping heart rate at 85 to 95 percent of your maximum. Cool down with 10 minutes of easy spinning in small chain ring at a heart rate of below 65 percent of maximum.

M	Tu	W	Th	F	Sa	Su
Run	Swim	Run	Bike	Rest	Swim	Bike
(Med.)	(Easy)	(Hard)	(Med.)		(Hard)	(Hard)
						Brick
						(Hard)

During the in-season phase, you can stop your lifting if you find it is making you sore and tired. You will lose very little of your strength while giving your body a better chance to recover and peak.

TRAINING PLAN

TAPER
[RACE WEEK]

One week

MONDAY

Run; medium run of 20 to 30 minutes at 65 to 75 percent of your maximum.

TUESDAY

Bike; easy 20- to 30-minute spin in small chain ring at a heart rate of 60 to 70 percent of your maximum.

WEDNESDAY

Swim; easy lap swimming for 10 to 15 minutes at 60 to 70 percent of maximum.

THURSDAY

Rest.

FRIDAY

Travel.

SATURDAY

Preview race course; note transition areas, difficult sections (i.e., hills, changes in running or riding surfaces, etc.).

SUNDAY

Race.

M	Tu	W	Th	F	Sa	Su
Run	Bike	Swim	Rest	Travel	Preview	Race
(Med.)	(Easy)	(Easy)			race course	

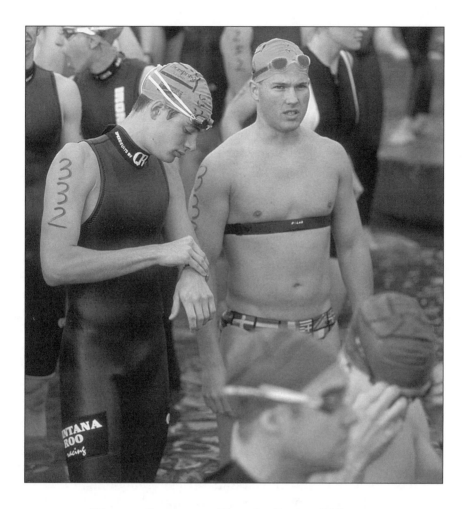

Keeping a Training Diary

Studies have shown that by recording various factors related to your training program, you help prevent the occurrence of problems such as overtraining. By writing down everything about your workouts, you can help chart trends that might negatively affect your training. Using a heart rate monitor is one way to make sure that you vary the intensity of your workouts to produce optimum results. In addition, factors such as hours of sleep, body weight, and an overall subjective stress/fatigue scale on which you rate how you feel from 1 to 10 have also been shown to help prevent overtraining and staleness.

Resting heart rate can be used as an indicator of how quickly you recover from your training sessions, in an effort to monitor overtraining. A general rule of thumb is that if there is more than a 5 to 10 beat per minute difference from one day to the next, there could be a problem, since your heart rate will usually go up when your body is fatigued. Finally, if writing down everything you do during training sounds boring, there are several software programs such as Ultra Coach, available for your home computer, that will make the process much easier.

Recovering From Exercise

Another essential ingredient that successful top athletes include in their training programs is the use of various methods for recovering from the stress of training and competing. One hot tip is to learn how to use your heart rate monitor to control your heart rate during and after a workout to help improve your running and cycling economy (or the ease at which you work out). This involves using a combination of deep "belly" breathing, visualization skills, positive self-talk, and progressive muscle relaxation. For more details, Polar has a brochure that explains the exact procedure. Based on research conducted by Dr. James Rippe, the Polar Take Ten Stress Reduction Program, as described in the brochure, is a simple but effective biofeedback process that helps reduce tension and fatigue. Other methods of speeding the recovery process from exercise include adequate amounts of sleep (about eight hours), proper nutrition and hydration, and whirlpool baths and massage, as well as active rest.

Symptoms of Overtraining

To help you pinpoint problems in your training schedule, I have developed a list of the symptoms of overtraining. You should think about using some of your recovery strategies if you find that you have any of these signs:

Increased perceived effort during your workout
Muscle and joint stiffness

Trouble finishing a workout
Extended recovery time after a workout
Increased rate of injury
Problems sleeping
Feelings of depression, anxiety, or anger
Low levels of energy
Weight loss
Constipation or diarrhea
Frequent illness
Decreased workout performance
Increased resting heart rate

Finally, If you do get a cold or some other illness, back off your training. Both colds and flu are caused by viruses that simply need time to run their course. So give yourself a break, and let your body do its job and get better. If you follow these basic rules, you can reach new heights of performance.

CHAPTER 8

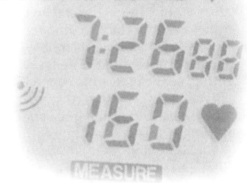

CIRCUIT TRAINING

WAYNE L. WESTCOTT

Every physical activity you do requires energy to power your muscles, which is provided by increased pumping action of the heart for an abundant supply of oxygen-rich blood. This is most easily observed by higher heart rates during and immediately after your exercise session.

There are essentially two energy systems that operate as you exercise. The aerobic energy system provides most of the energy during lower-intensity, longer-duration activities such as running or cycling. The anaerobic energy system provides most of the energy during higher-intensity, shorter-duration activities such as weight training and sprinting.

Both endurance exercise and strength exercise stimulate the heart to pump faster and harder, but the oxygen utilization is much higher during endurance exercise. This is so because endurance activities such as running involve many muscle groups that require lots of oxygen for energy production. The delivery system (heart) works hard and fast to pump oxygen-rich blood through the arteries and capillaries to the contracting muscles. The active receiving system (many muscle groups) extracts large amounts of oxygen from the blood.

On the other hand, strength exercise such as *circuit weight training* typically involves only one or two muscle groups at a time and therefore requires less energy. The delivery system (heart) pumps hard and fast to supply oxygen-rich blood to the working muscles, but the active receiving system (one or two muscle groups) extracts small to moderate amounts of oxygen from the blood. So endurance exercise and strength exercise produce similar responses in the delivery system but different responses in the receiving system, depending on the amount of muscle activated.

Circuit weight training is a conditioning program in which you perform one set of exercises for a given muscle group (e.g., quadriceps), followed closely by another set of exercises for a different muscle group (e.g., hamstrings), and so on for all the major muscle groups, typically 10 to 15 different exercises in close succession.

We know that aerobic exercise of sufficient intensity (60–85 percent of maximal heart rate), duration (20–60 minutes), and frequency (three to five days per week) is effective for improving our cardiovascular function, our ability to use oxygen, and our endurance performance, according to guidelines established by the American College of Sports Medicine in 1990. However, it is less clear whether circuit weight training is useful for cardiovascular conditioning. Although exercise studies reveal fewer cardiovascular adaptations from strength training than from endurance training, you may attain some cardiovascular benefits from a program of circuit strength training. Circuit weight training requires you to complete several different strength exercises with as little rest as possible between stations, thus maintaining a relatively high heart rate and cardiovascular effort.

On the positive side, research indicates that strength training may enhance cardiac muscle and increase the heart's pumping capacity. Studies also show that several weeks of circuit weight training may result in reduced resting blood pressure and lower levels of blood cholesterol. So, strength exercise seems to provide some cardiovascular benefits from a general health perspective, but let's take a closer look at the specific responses to circuit weight training.

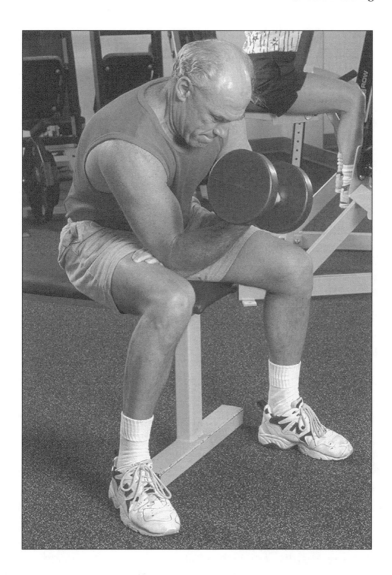

Cardiovascular Responses to Circuit Strength Training

What really takes place in the cardiovascular system during a circuit strength-training session? In a classic study by Hempel and Wells in 1985, 18 subjects were carefully monitored for heart rate and oxygen utilization as they performed a 14-station circuit of

Nautilus machines in a 20-minute time period. Each exercise was performed for 8 to 12 repetitions at about seven seconds per rep, in the following order:

1. Hip and back
2. Leg extension
3. Leg press
4. Leg curl
5. Calf raise
6. Pullover
7. Pulldown
8. Arm cross
9. Decline press
10. Lateral press
11. Overhead press
12. Biceps curl
13. Triceps extension
14. Abdominal

On average, the participants maintained an exercise heart rate of 143 beats per minute, which was about 75 percent of their maximal heart rate. However, their average exercise oxygen utilization was only 19 milliliters per kilogram per minute, just 37 percent of their maximal oxygen utilization ($\dot{V}O_2$max). The researchers concluded that circuit weight training produces a relatively high exercise heart rate but a relatively low oxygen utilization and is therefore only minimally effective for aerobic conditioning. Unfortunately, this study did not assess changes in cardiovascular fitness as a result of a circuit strength-training program. Let's examine some studies that did monitor the training outcomes.

Effect of Circuit Strength Training on Cardiovascular Performance

One of the key studies on the cardiovascular effects of circuit weight training was conducted in 1982 at the Cooper Institute for Aerobics Research. The 29 subjects completed three circuits of 10 strength exercises (Universal Gym weight-stack machines) in a 22.5-minute time period, taking only 15 seconds' rest between stations. After training three days a week for 12 weeks, the subjects' ability to use oxygen for endurance exercise ($\dot{V}O_2$max) increased by 12 percent.

Another important study on the cardiovascular effects of circuit weight training was conducted at Washington University School of Medicine in 1984. The 13 subjects performed one set of 14 Nautilus exercises, using 8 to 12 repetitions per set, taking about seven seconds per repetition and moving as quickly as possible between exercise stations. After training three days a week for 16 weeks, the participants' cardiovascular performance improved by 5 percent.

Perhaps the best-known circuit weight-training study was completed in 1985 at Wake Forest University. The 12 subjects performed one set of 12 Nautilus exercises using 8 to 12 repetitions for upper-body exercises and 15 to 20 repetitions for lower-body exercises. The training time was 20 minutes per session, and the training frequency was three days per week. After 10 weeks of circuit strength exercise, the trainees increased their ability to use oxygen by 11 percent. This significant improvement in cardiovascular performance was about equal to that experienced by a matched group of subjects who did 30 minutes of running, three days a week, during the same 10-week training period.

Why did similar circuit weight-training programs produce different results in cardiovascular performance? We're not sure, but the small number of research subjects may be partly responsible. In any case, these studies showed a 5 to 12 percent increase in the body's ability to use oxygen after circuit strength training, indicating a moderate degree of cardiovascular benefit.

During circuit strength training, the individual muscles work at a high effort level for about 1 to 2 minutes, but the heart works at a high effort level for about 20 minutes. Therefore, most of the aerobic improvements take place in the heart (delivery system) rather than in the muscles (receiving system). Because all the circuit weight-training studies showed major improvements in muscle strength, we could say that this type of exercise program benefits your muscular strength to a large extent and your cardiovascular endurance to a lesser extent, with little change in muscular endurance.

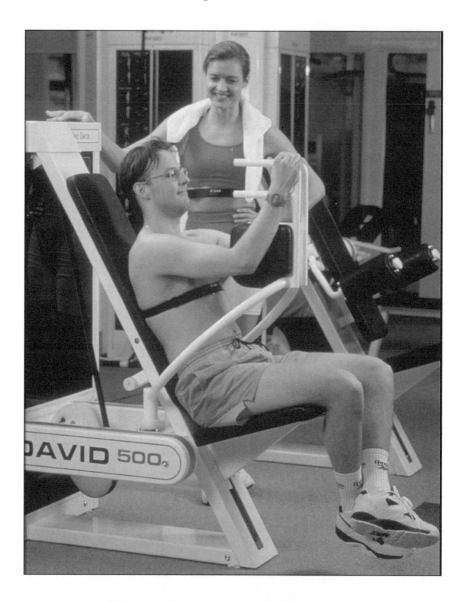

Practical Application

While the strength aspect of circuit weight training clearly exceeds the aerobic aspect, exercising in this manner may have certain advantages. To begin with, if you have limited training time, you can improve both your muscular and cardiovascular fitness in a 20-minute workout period.

Second, if you have injuries that temporarily restrict your aerobic activities, circuit weight training may be a practical exercise alternative. For example, after foot surgery I was unable to run, cycle, or swim, but I maintained my cardiovascular fitness through a regular program of circuit strength training.

Circuit weight training may also be used as a cross-training exercise in combination with other aerobic activities. For example, you could do cycling on Mondays, circuit strength training on Tuesdays, jogging on Thursdays, and circuit strength training on Fridays. This combination program provides training variety and places more equal emphasis on cardiovascular and muscular conditioning than performing only aerobic activities such as cycling, jogging, and stepping.

Guidelines for Heart Rate During Circuit Strength Training

Most of the research studies on circuit weight training produced exercise heart rates averaging about 75 percent of maximum. That is, if your maximal heart rate is 180 beats per minute, an effective circuit weight-training workout is likely to keep your heart rate around 135 beats per minute.

Of course, your heart rate will be lowest as you begin each exercise set and highest when you end each exercise set. For example, if your average training heart rate is 135 beats per minute, you may be as low as 120 beats per minute at the beginning of an exercise set and as high as 150 beats per minute at the end. The longer you rest between exercises, the longer you allow your heart to recover toward its resting rate. Generally speaking, healthy men and women should perform circuit weight training vigorously enough to maintain a heart rate response of about 70 to 80 percent of maximum.

Circuit strength training is also recommended for postcoronary patients as an effective and efficient means of physical conditioning. However, research indicates that lower training heart rates may be desirable. One study by Vander and co-workers of 21 cardiac patients showed that doing a circuit of Nautilus machines at about 55 to 65 percent of maximal heart rate produced no adverse effects. Another study by Kelemen and colleagues in 1986, with 20 cardiac patients, revealed no adverse responses to circuit weight-training workouts at about 75 percent of maximal heart rate. With physician approval, circuit weight-training exercise heart rates between 55 and 75 percent of maximum should be safe and productive for most postcoronary patients.

Recommended Weight Loads for Circuit Strength Training

Most of the studies on circuit strength training used approximately 75 percent of maximum resistance for the exercise weight loads. That is, if you can perform 1 repetition of an exercise with 100 pounds, you should use about 75 pounds for your circuit training weight load. Because most people can complete between 8 and 12 repetitions with 75 percent of maximum resistance, exercise weight loads that you can do for 10 repetitions should be just right for circuit strength training. You may train with less resistance if you prefer, but 75 percent of maximum weight load is recommended for best overall strength development.

Some circuit strength-training studies with postcoronary patients have used only 40 to 60 percent of maximum resistance, while others have shown excellent results with weight loads around 75 percent of maximum resistance. With their physicians' guidance, cardiac patients should probably begin circuit strength training with 40 to 60 percent of maximum resistance and gradually progress toward the 75 percent level.

Adjusting Intensity in Your Strength-Training Program

Your heart rate increases repetition by repetition as you perform a set of strength exercises. Therefore, one means for decreasing your heart rate response during circuit weight training is to perform fewer repetitions. For example, instead of doing 10 repetitions with 75 percent of your maximum resistance, you could end each set at 8 repetitions. Of course, you may also reduce the training intensity by using less resistance. Research I have conducted with colleagues shows that even a five-pound-lighter weight load can result in a lower cardiovascular response.

If you want to increase your heart rate, you may do the strength-training circuit more quickly, that is, taking shorter rests between successive exercises. In my own investigation of 30 subjects, completing the 10-station Nautilus circuit in 25 minutes resulted in an average heart rate of 128 beats per minute; finishing in 20 minutes produced an average heart rate of 139 beats per minute; and finishing in 15 minutes produced an average heart rate of 148 beats per minute.

Basically, circuit strength-training programs with shorter rest periods result in higher average heart rates, and circuit strength-training programs with longer rest periods result in lower average heart rates. For most practical purposes, your circuit strength-training rest periods should be less than 30 seconds. However, if you require a lower heart rate response, 60- to 90-second rest periods may be more suitable.

Monitoring Your Training Heart Rate

It is possible to palpate your pulse manually immediately before and after each set of strength exercises. However, because heart rates drop off quickly after the last repetition, manual pulse checks typically underestimate actual exercise heart rates. Because it is not possible to palpate your own pulse during the performance of most strength exercises, an electronic heart rate monitor may be useful.

Clearly, the best means for accurate and continuous heart rate recording during circuit weight training is using wireless and unobtrusive heart rate monitors. We have had greatest success with electronic devices that pick up the heart rate at the chest and provide a digital readout on a wrist monitor.

Once you have a heart rate monitor, use it regularly to provide performance feedback and enhance your circuit training benefits. Regular heart rate monitoring should enable you to exercise more consistently and productively, as well as help you to avoid inadvertently undertraining or overtraining.

The following are sample circuit strength-training programs for people interested in general fitness, for strength athletes, and for endurance athletes. As a general guideline, fitness enthusiasts and strength athletes should train at about 70 to 80 percent of maximal heart rate. Endurance athletes who have well-conditioned cardiovascular systems may prefer to train at a higher heart rate. Samples 1 and 2 present machine exercises and free-weight exercises for general

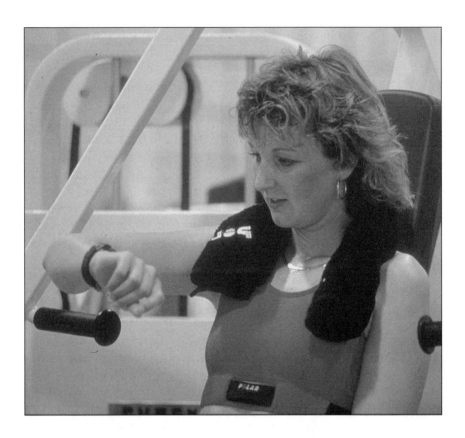

fitness. Samples 3 and 4 present machine exercises and free-weight exercises for strength athletes. Samples 5 and 6 present machine exercises and free-weight exercises for endurance athletes. The resistance machine exercises can be done in most fitness facilities; the free-weight exercises can be done in most fitness facilities or at home.

You should begin by doing just one circuit each workout. Use a resistance that will permit the recommended number of repetitions, performed with proper technique, through a full movement range, at about six seconds per repetition (two seconds lifting and four seconds lowering). Rest at least one day between exercise sessions.

As your cardiovascular system becomes better conditioned and one lap around the strength-training circuit feels less fatiguing, you may add a second lap to make your workout more challenging. Remember that your exercise form is a key factor in the success of your circuit strength-training program. Try to perform each exercise as if it were the only one you had to do, and you should see excellent results after just a few weeks of consistent training.

TRAINING PLAN

SAMPLE 1	Circuit Strength-Training Program for General Fitness: Machine Exercises

Exercise	Muscle group	Number of repetitions	Time for each exercise	Time between exercises
Leg extension	Quadriceps	8–12	50–70 sec	25–35 sec
Leg curl	Hamstrings	8–12	50–70 sec	25–35 sec
Leg press	Quadriceps, hamstrings	8–12	50–70 sec	25–35 sec
Chest cross	Chest	8–12	50–70 sec	25–35 sec
Pullover	Upper back	8–12	50–70 sec	25–35 sec
Lateral raise	Shoulders	8–12	50–70 sec	25–35 sec
Biceps curl	Biceps	8–12	50–70 sec	25–35 sec
Triceps extension	Triceps	8–12	50–70 sec	25–35 sec
Low back extension	Lower back	8–12	50–70 sec	25–35 sec
Abdominal curl	Abdominals	8–12	50–70 sec	25–35 sec
Neck flexion	Front neck	8–12	50–70 sec	25–35 sec
Neck extension	Rear neck	8–12	50–70 sec	25–35 sec

Total exercise for one circuit: 12

Total time for one circuit: about 18 minutes

Recommended heart rate: 70–80 percent of maximum

TRAINING PLAN

SAMPLE 2	Circuit Strength-Training Program for General Fitness: Free-Weight Exercises			
Exercise group repetitions	**Muscle of exercise**	**Number for each exercise**	**Time between**	**Time**
Dumbbell squat	Quadriceps, hamstrings	8–12	50–70 sec	25–35 sec
Dumbbell chest fly	Chest	8–12	50–70 sec	25–35 sec
Dumbbell lunge	Quadriceps, hamstrings	8–12	50–70 sec	25–35 sec
Dumbbell pullover	Upper back	8–12	50–70 sec	25–35 sec
Dumbbell calf raise	Calves	8–12	50–70 sec	25–35 sec
Dumbbell lateral raise	Shoulders	8–12	50–70 sec	25–35 sec
Dumbbell curl	Biceps	8–12	50–70 sec	25–35 sec
Dumbbell overhead extension	Triceps	8–12	50–70 sec	25–35 sec
Dumbbell shrug	Upper back, neck	8–12	50–70 sec	25–35 sec
Trunk curl	Abdominals	8–12	50–70 sec	25–35 sec
Back extension	Lower back	8–12	50–70 sec	25–35 sec

Total exercise for one circuit: 11

Total time for one circuit: about 16 minutes

Recommended heart rate: 70–80 percent of maximum

TRAINING PLAN

SAMPLE 3	**Circuit Strength-Training Program for Strength Athletes: Machine Exercises**

Exercise	Muscle group	Number of repetitions	Time for each exercise	Time between exercises
Hip adduction	Inner thigh	5–8	30–50 sec	35–45 sec
Hip abduction	Outer thigh	5–8	30–50 sec	35–45 sec
Leg press	Quadriceps, hamstrings	5–8	30–50 sec	35–45 sec
Chest press	Chest, triceps	5–8	30–50 sec	35–45 sec
Back row	Upper back, biceps	5–8	30–50 sec	35–45 sec
Shoulder press	Shoulders, triceps	5–8	30–50 sec	35–45 sec
Assisted chins	Upper back, biceps	5–8	30–50 sec	35–45 sec
Assisted dips	Chest, triceps	5–8	30–50 sec	35–45 sec
Biceps curl	Biceps	5–8	30–50 sec	35–45 sec
Triceps extension	Triceps	5–8	30–50 sec	35–45 sec
Low back extension	Lower back	5–8	30–50 sec	35–45 sec
Abdominal curl	Abdominals	5–8	30–50 sec	35–45 sec
Neck flexion	Front neck	5–8	30–50 sec	35–45 sec
Neck extension	Rear neck	5–8	30–50 sec	35–45 sec

Total exercise for one circuit: 14; Total time for one circuit: about 18 minutes; Recommended heart rate: 70–80 percent of maximum

TRAINING PLAN

SAMPLE 4	Circuit Strength-Training Program for Strength Athletes: Free-Weight Exercises			
Exercise	**Muscle group**	**Number of repetitions**	**Time for each exercise**	**Time between exercises**
Dumbbell squat	Quadriceps, hamstrings	5–8	30–50 sec	35–45 sec
Dumbbell chest fly	Chest, triceps	5–8	30–50 sec	35–45 sec
Dumbbell bent row	Upper back, biceps	5–8	30–50 sec	35–45 sec
Dumbbell shoulder press	Shoulders, triceps	5–8	30–50 sec	35–45 sec
Dumbbell lunge	Quadriceps, hamstrings	5–8	30–50 sec	35–45 sec
Dumbbell curl	Biceps	5–8	30–50 sec	35–45 sec
Dumbbell over-head extension	Triceps	5–8	30–50 sec	35–45 sec
Dumbbell upright row	Shoulders, neck	5–8	30–50 sec	35–45 sec
Dumbbell calf raise	Calves	5–8	30–50 sec	35–45 sec
Trunk curl	Abdominals	5–8	30–50 sec	35–45 sec
Back extension	Lower back	5–8	30–50 sec	35–45 sec

Total exercise for one circuit: 11

Total time for one circuit: about 15 minutes

Recommended heart rate: 70–80 percent of maximum

TRAINING PLAN

SAMPLE 5	Circuit Strength-Training Program for Endurance Athletes: Machine Exercises

Exercise	Muscle group	Number of repetitions	Time for each exercise	Time between exercises
Leg extension	Quadriceps	12–15	70–90 sec	15–25 sec
Leg curl	Hamstrings	12–15	70–90 sec	15–25 sec
Hip adduction	Inner thigh	12–15	70–90 sec	15–25 sec
Hip abduction	Outer thigh	12–15	70–90 sec	15–25 sec
Chest cross	Chest	12–15	70–90 sec	15–25 sec
Chest press	Chest and triceps	12–15	70–90 sec	15–25 sec
Pullover	Upper back	12–15	70–90 sec	15–25 sec
Back row	Upper back, biceps	12–15	70–90 sec	15–25 sec
Lateral raise	Shoulders	12–15	70–90 sec	15–25 sec
Shoulder press	Shoulders, triceps	12–15	70–90 sec	15–25 sec
Biceps curl	Biceps	12–15	70–90 sec	15–25 sec
Triceps extension	Triceps	12–15	70–90 sec	15–25 sec
Low back extension	Lower back	12–15	70–90 sec	15–25 sec
Abdominal curl	Abdominals	12–15	70–90 sec	15–25 sec
Neck flexion	Front neck	12–15	70–90 sec	15–25 sec
Neck extension	Rear neck	12–15	70–90 sec	15–25 sec

Total exercise for one circuit: 16; Total time for one circuit: about 27 minutes; Recommended heart rate: 75–85 percent of maximum

TRAINING PLAN

SAMPLE 6	Circuit Strength-Training Program for Endurance Athletes: Free-Weight Exercises

Exercise	Muscle group	Number of repetitions	Time for each exercise	Time between exercises
Dumbbell squat	Quadriceps, hamstrings	12–15	70–90 sec	15–25 sec
Dumbbell lunge	Quadriceps, hamstrings	12–15	70–90 sec	15–25 sec
Dumbbell calf raise	Calves	12–15	70–90 sec	15–25 sec
Dumbbell chest fly	Chest	12–15	70–90 sec	15–25 sec
Dumbbell chest press	Chest, triceps	2–15	70–90 sec	15–25 sec
Dumbbell pullover	Upper back	12–15	70–90 sec	15–25 sec
Dumbbell bent row	Upper back, biceps	12–15	70–90 sec	15–25 sec
Dumbbell lateral raise	Shoulders	12–15	70–90 sec	15–25 sec
Dumbbell shoulder press	Shoulders, triceps	12–15	70–90 sec	15–25 sec
Dumbbell curl	Biceps	12–15	70–90 sec	15–25 sec
Dumbbell over-head extension	Triceps	12–15	70–90 sec	15–25 sec
Dumbbell shrug	Upper back, neck	12–15	70–90 sec	15–25 sec
Trunk curl	Abdominals	12–15	70–90 sec	15–25 sec
Back extension	Lower back	12–15	70–90 sec	15–25 sec

Total exercise for one circuit: 14; Total time for one circuit: about 23 minutes; Recommended heart rate: 75–85 percent of maximum

CHAPTER 9

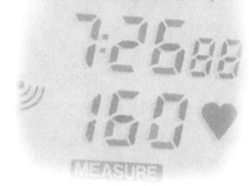

GROUP EXERCISE

JAY BLAHNIK

Group exercise is quite simply defined as working out in a group, led by an instructor, with the use of music. In the early 1980s, dance studios all over the country began offering these new exercise classes as a part of their regular dance class schedules. Slowly people became excited about this new workout form and the enthusiasm began to spread. One actress and ex-dancer was so excited about the new exercise format that she opened one of the very first studios to exclusively offer group exercise classes to the public—the Jane Fonda Workout Studio in Los Angeles, California. Fonda thought others who had not tried this new workout form would like it as much as she did, so she decided to produce a home workout video of her favorite class. No one, including Jane, realized the impact that first video would have on the newly born fitness industry. Millions of copies of the video were sold, and group exercise went from virtual obscurity to mainstream America almost overnight.

This form of exercise has evolved into a variety of sophisticated class formats since it first appeared in dance studios. Group exercise classes are an integral part of almost every gym and fitness center around the world. Many types of formats for group exercise classes have been created to offer variety and to attract all fitness levels and interests. You can select from high/low impact and step aerobics to muscle conditioning, circuit training, and indoor cycling. The choices are endless! With the wide variety of classes available, it is now easier and more appealing for anyone to work out in a class setting. Even men, who were not traditionally interested in these classes, now participate in record numbers.

What other factors make group exercise so popular? When you look at the multitude of benefits, it is easy to see why so many people enjoy participating on a regular basis.

- **Qualified fitness instructors.** Most classes are led by trained instructors who have been educated on how to lead large groups of people through safe and invigorating workouts.

- **Music.** Group exercise classes almost always include some form of music. Music can serve as a positive and motivating force for people to exercise. Studies have shown that people enjoy exercise more, perceive it to be less difficult, and may work out harder when they incorporate music with their workout.

- **Social interaction.** Group exercise classes provide a great environment for meeting people and enjoying social interaction. Larger classes may have as many as 50–100 people, while smaller classes may have only 5–20 people. Either way, you have the opportunity to be with other individuals who share a similar interest in working out.

- **Motivation.** Many people find that working out in a group setting motivates them to adhere to their exercise program. Setting a regular class schedule for yourself helps to create an enjoyable and rewarding fitness routine.

- **Variety.** With so many different group exercise class formats available, you can literally work out every day without taking the same type of workout or having the same instructors. This variety can reduce the risk of injury, prevent boredom, and keep you motivated.

- **Comprehensiveness.** Most important, group exercise classes are comprehensive, providing you with a thorough and complete workout. At the very least, most classes include warm-up, cool-down, and stretch segments. In addition, some classes even provide the opportunity to perform other unique activities such as stress reduction. All in 60 minutes or less!

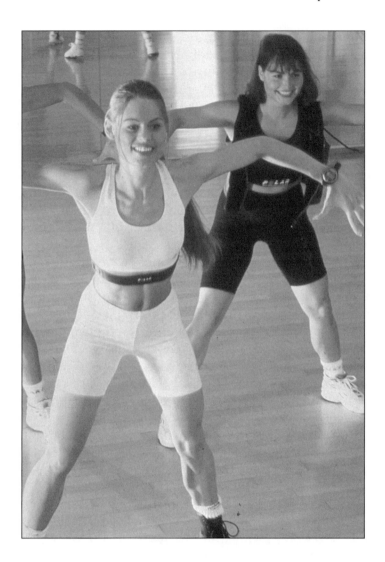

Using Heart Rate Monitors in Group Exercise

Proper exercise monitoring is extremely important in order for you to get results from any workout. However, group exercise classes pose some unique challenges to monitoring your intensity. Without a heart rate monitor, you have only two ways to monitor yourself in a group exercise setting—through perceived exertion or pulse palpation.

Unfortunately, as we have learned, these methods are usually not very accurate because of miscounting, miscalculating, and misinterpreting exertion level. Group exercise classes are no exception.

For example, many group exercise classes follow a routine, or perform choreography, that uses the arms and requires the class to move together. This makes it difficult to count the pulse rate without completely stopping the activity. It not only breaks up the flow and energy of the class; it also causes the heart rate to drop (which will then give you an inaccurate reading). The choreography in a group exercise class also requires a certain amount of mental concentration for safe and correct execution. Therefore, unless the instructor stops the routine, it is difficult to think clearly about your own perceived exertion.

Furthermore, there is a certain amount of energy and adrenaline that is created when people work out together. This is one of the best benefits of group exercise; it is highly motivating. However, performing the choreography with dynamic music playing can take your attention away from your breathing rate and the amount of power you are using to perform each movement. This can make it difficult to determine, through perceived exertion, how hard you are actually working. Some days you may not be working very hard, but the music and the excitement of the routine or choreography can make you feel as if you are working much harder than you actually are.

Finally, you may find yourself using the instructor's or other participants' workout intensity as a "benchmark" for how hard you should be working, even if their fitness level is different from yours. For example, working out next to a student who is less fit that you may cause you not to work as hard as you could. You might perceive your intensity to be lower than it is because that particular student lacks the stamina and energy that you have. Conversely, taking a class with an instructor who is extremely fit and works out very hard when he or she teaches may cause you to believe that you are working out harder than you actually are.

Finding Your Optimal Training Intensity for Group Exercise

A heart rate monitor can eliminate many of the challenges you will find in monitoring your intensity in a group exercise setting.

A heart rate monitor allows you to check your heart rate as frequently as you desire. There is no need to stop your activity, interrupt the choreography, or disrupt the other students. Most important, your heart rate will not drop while you are checking your pulse rate.

Additionally, you will not be misled by the energy and adrenaline that is created by working out side by side with other people. The music may be high energy, the participants may be shouting, and you may feel fantastic, but your heart rate monitor will allow you to accurately assess whether you need to be working harder or easier, regardless of these external motivators. If you are attempting to keep up with the person next to you, a heart rate monitor will allow you to determine whether that intensity is correct for you.

Getting Started

Before we review how you can best utilize your heart rate monitor in various types of group exercise classes, it is important for you to determine what type of class or classes are best for you. By doing this, you will increase your chances of reaching your workout and fitness goals.

What Do You Enjoy?

Think about what type of activity you like. If you have always enjoyed swimming, or being in the water, you might want to try water fitness classes. If you love to dance, you might want to try a traditional aerobics class or funky hip-hop exercise class. If you have a more athletic background, then circuit training or interval training may be best for you.

Do Your Homework

Observe a class before you decide to take it, if you are unsure of the format. By doing this you can see whether the activity looks like fun and whether it would be a good match for your interests and experience. Be sure to read the class description and perhaps ask other students their opinions of each class. Usually you can get a good idea of what you are getting yourself into by doing a little

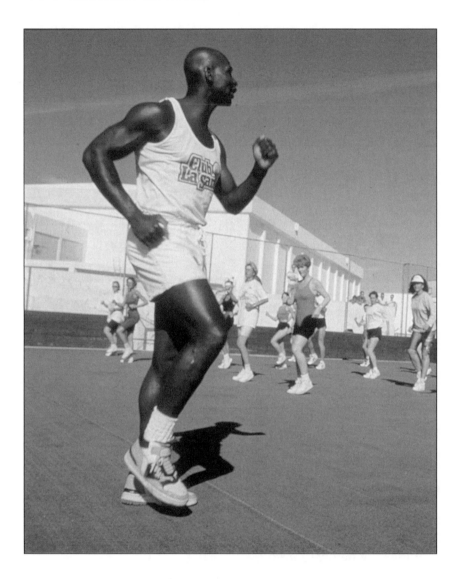

homework. The last thing you want is to go to a class that is an unnatural match for your skills and interests.

Determine Your Skill Level

You should honestly evaluate your coordination and agility. Some group exercise classes require you to learn complicated foot and arm patterns as part of the routine. While these types of classes can be fun, they can also be frustrating if you are unable to keep pace with the other participants. Try to select a class in which the coordination requirements match your skills. This will improve your chances for success and increase your enjoyment of the class. Once you have mastered certain coordination skills, you can try other classes to challenge yourself.

What Kind of Results Are You Looking For?

Finally, you should determine what kind of results you are seeking before you choose your class. For example, if you are looking to lose weight and/or body fat and improve your cardiovascular fitness, you should choose a class that has a significant aerobic training component (i.e., high/low impact aerobics, step aerobics, or interval training). If you want to improve your muscular strength or tone up, you might find circuit training or muscular conditioning classes a better match. Usually you will find that a combination of classes works best; but for maximum benefit, you should participate in classes that get you the desired results. This will ensure that you stay active for life!

Designing Your Group Exercise Program

Unlike cycling, running, or in-line skating, group exercise is not characterized by one type of activity. Group exercise classes come in many different formats, each of which has a definite focus. The three main categories for group exercise classes are cardiovascular conditioning, muscular conditioning, and flexibility/stress reduction. Let us take a closer look at each of these categories.

Cardiovascular Conditioning

Cardiovascular conditioning classes are specifically designed to make the heart and lungs stronger and improve body composition through aerobic activity. This is achieved by using the large muscles of the lower body in continuous rhythmic movement. There are two types of cardiovascular conditioning classes: steady state and interval training. While working in steady state, the heart rate is elevated to a determined level, usually between zone 2 and zone 4 (see table 9.1, intensity classification chart, which is maintained for a period of time. A heart rate monitor is essential with steady state training, as it allows you to watch your workout carefully and stay within these zones. Interval training is characterized by bouts of intense activity (usually in zone 4 or zone 5), alternated with periods of less intense activity (usually in zone 1 or zone 2) designed for heart rate recovery. With interval training, a heart rate monitor is a valuable tool to use to ensure that you are attaining specific heart rates for both the intense segments and the recovery phases. You will experience the most significant heart rate response with both of these types of cardiovascular conditioning classes as compared to classes that focus on muscular conditioning or flexibility.

The various types of cardiovascular conditioning classes include the following:

■ **High/low impact aerobics.** Participants perform high-impact (i.e., running) and low-impact (i.e., marching) athletic and dance-based movements. Generally, no equipment or exercise tools are required.

■ **Step aerobics.** Participants perform athletic and dance-based movements on and off of an adjustable platform. This type of class usually provides a more intense lower-body workout.

■ **Slide aerobics.** Participants slide side to side on a specially designed slide board, mimicking activities such as skating and

TABLE 9.1 Group Exercise Intensity Classifications by Zone

Training zone	RPE	Used for	Percent MHR
Zone 1	Very easy	Recovery	50–60
Zone 2	Easy	Endurance (warm-up)	60–70
Zone 3	Moderate	Stamina	70–80
Zone 4	Hard	Performance	80–90
Zone 5	Very hard	Maximum	90–100

skiing. This type of class provides an intense workout for the muscles that make up the inner and outer thighs.

■ **Aerobic circuit training.** Participants perform a variety of cardiovascular conditioning activities at specific stations set up around a room. Participants generally work in small groups or individually.

■ **Dance-based aerobics.** Participants perform specific dance routines based on country line dancing, hip-hop, funk, and other types of dance. This type of class usually involves complex arm and foot patterns.

■ **Indoor cycling.** Participants engage in a simulated outdoor all-terrain cycling journey on a specially designed stationary cycle. This type of class allows the participant to focus on achieving personal performance and fitness goals while training to become a better cyclist.

■ **Water fitness.** Participants perform a variety of athletic and dance-based movements in the water. Because the body is naturally buoyant in the water, this type of class reduces the impact forces to the skeletal system.

Muscular Conditioning

Muscular conditioning classes are specifically designed to make muscles stronger through the use of weights and/or resistance tools such as elastic bands and tubing. Generally speaking, muscular conditioning classes do not provide as high a heart rate response as cardiovascular conditioning classes (usually between zone 1 and zone 2). However, within the framework of a muscular conditioning class, you will notice that lower-body exercises, such as lunges and squats, will elicit a higher heart rate response than upper-body exercises. (Remember, the larger the muscle groups involved in a given activity, the higher the heart rate response will be.)

The various types of muscular conditioning classes include the following:

■ **Body sculpting.** Participants perform series of exercises, as a group, to strengthen specific parts of the body or the entire body.

■ **Muscular conditioning circuit training.** Participants perform muscular conditioning activities at specific stations set up around the room. They generally work in small groups or individually.

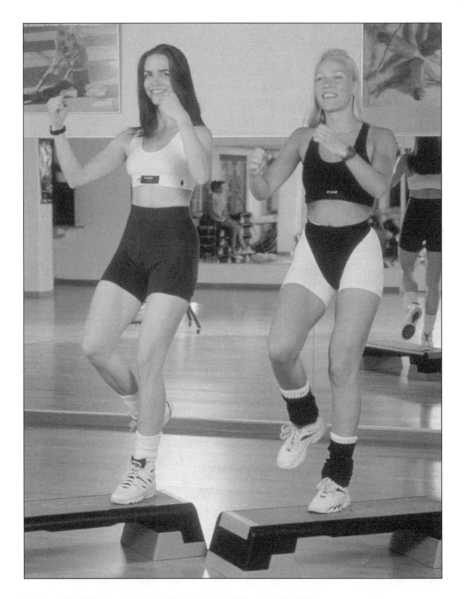

Flexibility and Stress Reduction

Flexibility and stress reduction classes are designed to increase range of motion and flexibility while teaching you how to reduce and manage stress. These types of classes will provide you with a lower heart rate response than cardiovascular and muscular conditioning classes (usually in zone 1). In fact, lowering the heart rate is often a specific goal of these types of classes.

The various types of flexibility and stress reduction classes include the following:

■ **Stretch.** Participants perform static athletic movements designed to improve range of motion and flexibility. Although special techniques are not usually employed to lower the heart rate, the static nature of these movements will naturally result in a lower heart rate response.

■ **Yoga.** Participants perform a sequence of static poses with special attention to breathing techniques, all designed to increase flexibility, balance, and coordination. Many of the poses can be athletic and intense enough to elevate the heart rate significantly when compared to the movements performed in traditional stretch classes (sometimes as high as zone 3).

■ **Tai chi.** Participants perform a sequence of dynamic, fluid poses designed to improve mental concentration and serenity. Because of tai chi's continuous rhythmic movements, the lower heart rate response tends to remain steady, with a very small amount of variation.

■ **Guided imagery and biofeedback.** Participants engage in a meditative, auditory experience that involves little or no movement. Because of the relaxing nature of the imagery, heart rate response tends to remain low and steady.

As you design your individual group exercise program, it is important to evaluate your heart rate response in relation to your interests, skills, fitness level, and most important, your goals. Selecting classes that will give you the opportunity to reach your specific goals is essential for success and will help you to train more efficiently and effectively.

Sample Workout Schedule—Multiclass Format

You could utilize this sample workout schedule if you enjoy a variety of types of classes and want to improve your fitness level. This particular schedule incorporates high/low impact, step, and indoor cycling classes. You can replace any of these three types of classes with another type of class such as slide or circuit training, if you wish. Please note that the time durations listed do not include warm-up and cool-down.

TRAINING PLAN

Multiclass Format Workout Schedule

Day	Type of class	Zone	Goal	Duration
Monday	High/Low impact	3	Stamina	40 minutes
Tuesday	Step	2	Endurance	40–50 minutes
Wednesday	Indoor	4 and 1 cycling	Performance (intervals)	30 minutes
Thursday	Rest			
Friday	High/Low impact	2	Endurance	40–50 minutes
Saturday	Step	3	Stamina	40 minutes
Sunday	Rest			

Sample Workout Schedule— Single-Class Format

This sample workout schedule would be appropriate for you if you enjoy participating in only one type of class format and want to improve your fitness level. Step aerobics is used in this example; however, for step you can substitute other types of classes such as high/low impact aerobics or indoor cycling, if desired. Please note that the time durations listed do not include warm-up and cool-down.

Adjusting Intensity in Your Group Exercise Classes

Generally speaking, the more energy and muscle that you put into any activity, the more challenging it will be. Therefore, the best way

▮ TRAINING PLAN

Single-Class Format Workout Schedule

Day	Type of class	Zone	Goal	Duration
Monday	Step	4 and 1 (intervals)	Performance	35 minutes
Tuesday	Step	2	Endurance	45–50 minutes
Wednesday	Step	3	Stamina	40 minutes
Thursday	Step	2	Endurance	45–50 minutes
Friday	Rest			
Saturday	Step	4 and 1 (intervals)	Performance	35 minutes
Sunday	Rest			

to modify your intensity is to manipulate how hard you work. In a group exercise class, you can modify only to a point that still allows you to participate with the rest of the group. In other words, in contrast to the situation in individual sports, you cannot just do your own thing.

Keeping this in mind, let us look at some ways you can modify your movements during each type of class to make the activity more or less intense.

Cardiovascular Conditioning Classes

■ **High/low impact aerobics.** If you want to make this type of class more challenging, you might choose to jump a little higher when doing kicks or knee lifts. You could also bend your knees more when doing movements like jumping jacks or step touches. Finally, try pumping the arms more vigorously while marching or jogging. Conversely, if you need to make the workout less challenging, do smaller leg movements and eliminate the arm movements.

■ **Step aerobics.** The easiest way to make this type of class more challenging is to increase the height of your step platform, which will make all your movements more strenuous. You can also try adding hops or jumps to the more traditional, basic step moves. To make this format less challenging, simply reduce the height of your step platform or eliminate the hops and jumps.

■ **Slide aerobics.** You will likely find this type of class plenty challenging because it requires explosive, powerful leg movements. If necessary, however, you can make it more challenging by sliding across the board with a "lower profile" (i.e., dropping closer to the board by bending your knees more and not letting your feet come together at the end of each slide across). You could also do a "speed slide" by executing three quick slides across in the same amount of time you might normally do just two slides across. Conversely, you might try taking a longer pause between each slide across if you want to make the workout less challenging.

■ **Aerobic circuit training.** In this type of class, you can decrease your overall intensity by doing the most challenging cardio-vascular stations a little bit more slowly, or you can increase your overall intensity by doing the easier stations a little more vigorously.

■ **Dance-based aerobics.** Since this type of class usually involves complex arm and foot patterns, the mental challenge may often be greater than the physical challenge. If you find you need to make the workout more intense, try eliminating the arm patterns from the routine until you can comfortably do the foot patterns more vigorously. Then add the arm patterns back into the routine.

■ **Indoor cycling.** You can easily decrease the intensity in this type of workout by slowing down your revolutions per minute, lessening the amount of tension on the flywheel, or sitting down during the drills that are normally done in a more aggressive, standing position.

■ **Water fitness.** You can make a water workout more challenging by following the same guidelines as for a high/low aerobics class, or by moving faster through the water, which will provide resistance against your movements. If you want to make the workout less challenging, try making your movements smaller so that you will not have to move as quickly through the water while doing the specified routine or movements.

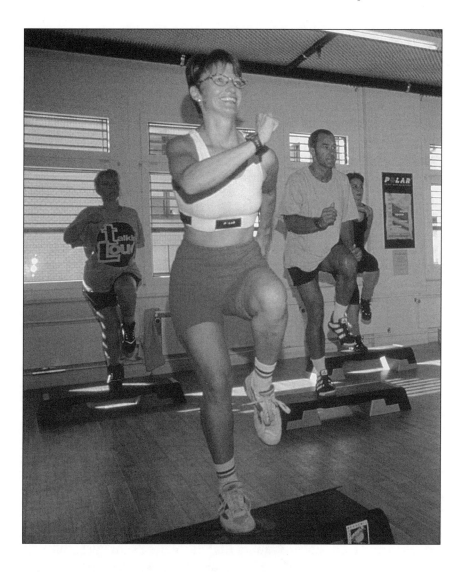

Muscular Conditioning Classes

■ **Body sculpting.** If your heart rate is elevated higher than you would like, then it may be necessary to do fewer repetitions or to use a lighter weight. For example, if you are doing a set of lunges with weights, and you feel you must stop because you are becoming winded, you could put the weights down and then finish the set. Over time, as you become stronger, you will be able to complete the set with the weights and achieve your desired heart rate response.

■ **Muscular conditioning circuit training.** In this type of class, you can decrease your overall intensity by using less weight (or no weight) at the circuit stations that you find particularly challenging or by doing the exercises a little bit more slowly and less vigorously. You can increase your overall intensity by using heavier weights and executing the lower-body exercise stations with greater intensity. Remember, the stations that utilize the smaller, upper-body muscles will not elicit as high a heart rate response as those stations that target the lower body.

Flexibility and Stress Reduction Classes

■ **Stretch.** As already mentioned, most traditional stretches will not elicit a high heart rate response; however, stretches that require you to balance or stabilize the weight of your body might cause the heart rate to increase due to the isometric contractions involved. If this is the case, use the wall, a bench, or a bar to support yourself and reduce the need to balance and stabilize the body. Also, remember to breathe deeply and evenly during all stretches. Holding your breath can increase your blood pressure, which can result in a higher heart rate response.

■ **Yoga.** If you find that a particular yoga sequence is too challenging, you could simply come out of the pose sooner. If you are in a position closer to the floor, you could release to a kneeling resting position; if you are in a more upright pose, you could relax in a standing position. You can also check with the instructor for more specific recommendations.

■ **Tai chi.** The fluid nature of tai chi tends to elicit a low, steady heart rate response. However, some tai chi movements require you to perform small dips or squats that can cause some variability in your heart rate. To reduce this variability, simply decrease the width of your leg stance and make your dip and squat movements smaller.

■ **Guided imagery and biofeedback.** One of the main objectives of this type of class is to reduce the heart rate. You will find it easier to accomplish this goal if you establish a breathing pattern that is deep and steady. In addition, blocking out external distractions such as noise or light by focusing your attention and/or shutting your eyes will also help to reduce your heart rate. If you are distracted or unfocused, you will usually see a higher heart rate response.

Taking Your Group Exercise Training to a Higher Level

Once you have worked with your program or activity for a while, you will notice that it will become less challenging overall. If you want to continue to make gains and become stronger, you will need to push yourself beyond what you have become accustomed to. Let's discuss how to modify your program so that you can make it more challenging.

■ **Pick a specific amount of time during which you will increase the heart rate to a level higher than usual.** For example, spend five minutes at 148 beats per minute versus your normal rate of 143 beats per minute. Then, slowly increase the amount of time that you spend at this higher heart rate. Watch your heart rate monitor to track this.

■ **Take a class that has a longer format or involves more work.** For example, select an advanced step class versus the intermediate one that you have attended for months. Remember, in this particular case you are not trying to get your heart rate higher; you are simply trying to sustain your heart rate in the desired training zone for a longer period of time.

■ **Switch activities.** If you tend to take only step or slide classes, try doing a water fitness class. Your body will be forced to use the cardiovascular system and muscles in ways they are not utilized in step or slide classes. This will be evident as you monitor your heart rate response.

■ **Add a day or a class.** If you normally work out three times per week, try increasing your workout schedule to four times per week or, if your schedule permits, take one type of class in the morning and a different type in the evening. Be aware of your heart rate response and possible signs of overtraining.

Conclusion

Group exercise has come a long way from its humble beginnings in the early 1980s. Group exercise has evolved to form the heart and soul of many fitness programs in gyms and fitness centers around the world. Millions of individuals participate every day, in a variety of classes, to experience the music, energy, and camaraderie unique to this form of activity.

We now have the technology to monitor this form of exercise to ensure that it is both efficient and effective. Although it is easy to get distracted with the music, choreography, and adrenaline present in most group exercise classes, accurately assessing your intensity level has never been easier. Heart rate monitors allow us to carefully track our heart rate response in our group exercise workouts. Whether you are taking a step class, a body-sculpting class, or an indoor cycling class, you can observe your individual heart rate response to ensure that you are training within your determined target zone. A heart rate monitor allows you to stay both focused and motivated to help you reach your fitness goals.

Remember, take time to assess which types of group exercise classes you will enjoy most. By selecting classes that will be a good match for your fitness level, coordination, and fitness goals, you will ensure success in reaching those goals. Track your heart rate response in all the classes you participate in, as this will enable you to determine which classes are best for you.

To adjust intensity in your group exercise classes, don't overlook the obvious: The more energy you put into a given class, the more challenging it will be. Observe your individual heart rate response and modify your activity accordingly. To make your workout more rigorous, you may choose to jump a little higher, add height to your step platform, or increase the amount of weight with which you are working. To decrease the intensity of your workout, simply lighten the load of that specific activity. By keeping an eye on your heart rate monitor, you will be able to personally tailor your workout to your specific needs within the framework of any class.

Lastly, keep in mind that varying your exercise routine is essential for success. If you find that you are not as challenged by a group exercise class as you were at the beginning, consider these additional suggestions. *Switch activities.* If you have been attending the same step or slide class for six months, try adding some weight training to your program. The strength you will gain with your weight training will have an added benefit—that of making it easier for you to work harder in your other group exercise classes. *Add a day.* Try going from three days a week to four or five days per week. *Take a class that involves more work.* You may choose a class that has a longer format or involves other fitness components not offered in the classes you normally attend. By monitoring your heart rate response, it will be easy to tell whether or not you are truly challenging yourself.

Experience what a difference the use of a heart rate monitor can make in a group exercise setting. Set yourself up for success by carefully tracking your heart rate response to the activities you enjoy most. You will find that you are working more efficiently and effectively to reach your fitness goals.

CHAPTER 10

MONITORING THE TRAINING EFFECT

JIM DOTTER

By now it should be clear that continuously monitoring your heart's response to a workout, and having this immediate feedback during the workout, can facilitate intelligent choices and a controlled, systematic approach to the workout. This information, now highly accurate and accessible, marks the difference between a workout that advances you toward your goal and one that serves no purpose, or worse, causes damage and nullifies the gains you had purchased by months of prior effort.

But what about feedback on the long term, as you adjust your training plan through the season? You can apply the same principles of awareness, control, and intelligent choices to your training over calendar time—choosing the right workouts and the right effort level and reacting to the changes that occur as your body responds to training. Just as during the workout, the key is to get and maintain accurate information in an accessible, understandable form without spending too much time gathering it.

With the addition of a heart rate monitor, you have a terrific new tool for long-term planning and analysis. This chapter will present some techniques for using that new tool to put together a program for success, however you choose to measure it.

The Keys to Success: Planning, Logging, and Analysis

The degree to which your training effort results in improvement depends on the structure and organization you apply to it. A workout is not an isolated event; it should be part of an overall plan, designed for a purpose. Top athletes and coaches know this, and their training management can be divided into three parts: planning, logging, and analysis. Even if your goals are less ambitious, you will still benefit from giving a small amount of time to each of these.

Planning

It is important to make a plan and commit it to writing or to your computer. Besides the obvious need to remember what the plan was in order to follow it for a number of weeks or months, there is a psychological need to make the commitment and see it through. There are important physiological reasons as well.

Most coaches agree that a steady state approach to fitness training is not productive. Trying to maintain the highest possible fitness level on a permanent basis leads to overtraining. Also, a steady state of effort at a lower level becomes ineffective because the body adapts to that level and then stops developing. Because of this, running the same three-mile loop, for example, at the same pace, day in and day out, quickly reaches a point of diminishing returns.

A good plan has a structure that fluctuates through periods of greater and lesser effort, to keep the body from settling into stasis at a given fitness level and to keep our ambitions from leading us into overstress and injury. A coach designs these phases or cycles of training in order to lead the athlete to a performance peak at a certain time. The athlete could not maintain that level for long, but derives a psychological boost (or fame and fortune) from a good performance. In the long term, this approach develops the athlete without injury, so that next year's peak will be higher than this year's. Your own training plan will be more effective if it involves this type of phased approach, or at least some fluctuations in the training effort from week to week. This requires long-term planning.

With heart rate-based training, you have some exciting new options in planning your training. You can specify the target training zone for each workout, or an effort range that you translate to a heart rate range when you are ready to perform the workout. And you can quantify the amount of training you will do at different zones in the different phases of your plan.

Logging

Keeping a good record of what you've done in training is essential because it sets you up for the third key, which is analysis and adjustment. If you have no record of what you've been doing, it is difficult to make intelligent adjustments. Consistency is most important. If you keep just a few facts but keep them consistently, every workout, you'll have grist for later study. A lot of data one week, followed by a blank sheet the next, makes a difficult mix from which to derive any understanding.

It is not necessary to spend a lot of time keeping records if you record only the information you will really want later. If a particular piece of information offers no insight when you are ready for the analysis part, don't save it. The key is to know what information you'll want later and to be sure to gather that consistently. Further on in this chapter, I'll show you several approaches to logging data, with different levels of detail. You'll find that if you are organized, you can log enough information for a good analysis in just a couple of minutes a day.

Analysis

Once you have a good plan, and after you have followed the plan for a time and have kept good records, you'll be ready for the most productive, interesting, and enjoyable part of the whole process: analyzing your response to the training. Over time, you'll learn what works for you and what mistakes to avoid. After a while you'll be getting more improvement out of the same amount of time and effort and will have fewer setbacks from injury or burnout. The key is to set up for this analysis in the way you make your plan and in your system for keeping records. I will show you some ways you can get set up for planning, logging, and analysis in the context of heart rate training, ranging from simple to fairly sophisticated.

The best way to find meaning in the numbers is to look for a cause-and-effect relationship. This is best done by comparing what you have done (your training data) to the progress you've made (evaluation). Another component that can add to the picture is changes to your personal "barometers" (body weight, resting heart rate, etc.). The best way is to look at all three of these components together, objectively measured and preferably displayed in a graphical form, as shown in figure 10.1. Having the three graphs, stacked one above the next, all with the same calendar time along the bottom axis, helps you see and understand the cause-and-effect relationships and eventually learn to manage them. It sounds like something from a degree program in exercise physiology, but it is really very simple to do, and very rewarding.

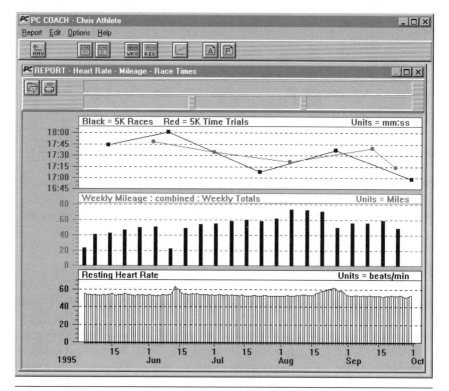

Figure 10.1   Graphs showing workout performance data, performance evaluations, and personal stats.

Tools

Before you decide on an approach to training management, make a list of the tools you will have for gathering data, for guiding your workout, and for recording and analyzing. These include your heart monitor (be sure you know what data it records and reports), a sport watch if these functions are not included in your monitor, a bike speedometer, a pool clock, built-in electronics on exercise machines—all the things you have that can report objective, numeric data about your workout. For recording and analyzing, you may have access to a computer or may use pen and paper. If the latter, be aware of the time required for detailed tracking and consider a less ambitious approach to data gathering.

The system you create depends largely on the tools you have for gathering data. The better the tools, the better your program can be, assuming you put a little thought into how to use them. Misapplied, high-tech tools add nothing to the picture. Also, different models of heart monitors allow for different possibilities in data logging and analysis. A model that reports only elapsed time and average heart rate dictates a limited approach to record keeping. While elapsed time is good, warm-up and cool-down time skews the reported average heart rate, so you must be careful about when you start the monitor if you want to track your time in the zone. A better model of monitor that reports the time spent within a certain zone, or above a low threshold (nearly the same thing), makes "time in zone" a practical option. If you have this feature, it can be included in your logging system.

More advanced models of heart monitors record lap times or split times as well as heart rates. These offer a convenient, integrated tool and eliminate the need to wear a sport watch on the other wrist during races and interval workouts. Either way, lap and split times can be added to your data-gathering system to good effect.

Finally, for users who like the details, there are advanced heart monitor models that record a heart rate profile throughout the entire workout. Further, take advantage of the ability to download this information to the computer. It is worth noting that such a system, including the necessary computer software, is now affordable for most individuals (fig. 10.2). Indicative of the revolutionary changes occurring in sport training, information of this quality—now available to everyone—was beyond the reach of most professional exercise physiologists 15 years ago.

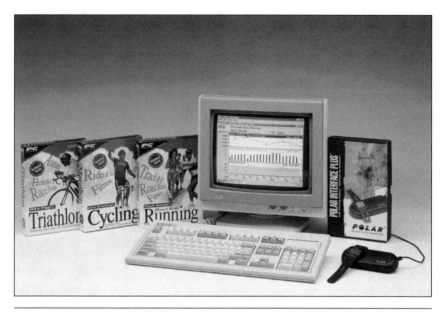

Figure 10.2 A training system integrating heart rate monitor, computer, and training software.

The Importance of Software

If you have access to a personal computer, there are tremendous advantages to using it as a training management tool. This is true whether or not you plan to download the data directly from your heart monitor. The power and flexibility of the computer are useful in all three phases: planning, logging, and especially analysis, where the ability to see your data graphically displayed can help you identify trends. A graphical view can make cause-and-effect relationships between your plan and your improvement obvious. You could use a standard spreadsheet program, but I recommend a more specialized tool. Affordable sport training software, such as the PC Coach software training system or the Polar Training Advisor, provides excellent tools for planning, logging, and analysis all in one integrated package.

If you are looking for help in setting up a program, software packages by several well-known authors, including Dr. Edmund Burke and Roy Benson, are available that are specifically designed for heart rate training. These packages set up the structural framework and the specific workout recommendations you need and give you access to a wealth of heart rate coaching knowledge.

What to Look for in a Software Package

Choosing the software you will use as your logbook is an important step, deserving of a little attention. Once you've started with one package, it is often impossible to get data from that system imported into a package of a different brand. Here are some things to consider when selecting your foundation software tool:

■ **The ability to plan ahead.** You should be able to put workouts on your calendar on future days, with goal data included, and then enter actual data when that day arrives.

■ **Flexible logging capabilities.** Look for a package that gives you the power to decide what data to log, rather than giving you a fixed set of fields that you can't change. The software should include a tool with which you can create your own custom workouts, with any amount and type of data.

■ **Graphical representations of any data.** Following from the last item, if you store a piece of information you should be able to graph it out.

■ **A coaching option.** Look for a package that offers more than just a logbook function. You might want to plug in a software coaching option at some point and let it guide you in setting up your plan. Be sure that the package tells you whose coaching advice you are following and also make sure that the person is a knowledgeable coach or expert, not just the computer programmer.

■ **Compatibility.** The software you choose should be compatible with your heart rate monitor. For monitors that download, be sure the data link in directly without requiring you to perform the download operation a second time. For non-downloading models, be sure that the software is flexible enough to store the information your monitor (and other equipment) reports.

■ **Support.** Look for free technical support, preferably with a toll-free number. Also, expect a money-back satisfaction guarantee. You can be pretty sure that a company that stands by its product in this way is delivering quality merchandise. Check to be sure that the company has been in this business for several years. See whether the company's web site is aimed solely at sales or whether there is a support area too, with an FAQ ("frequently asked questions") page. Ask about the documentation that comes with the product.

Determining the Essential Information for Your Training System

There are three categories of data that you can include when setting up your program: training data, performance evaluations, and personal "stats" that act as indicators of change in your body. While training data are useful in both planning and logging, as in "planned versus actuals," evaluations and stats are only logged. If you can record something from each of these three categories, even something simple, then you'll have a good start on a useful program. In the following paragraphs, each category is treated separately.

Training Data

Typically a coach sets up a training plan based on two abstractions: training volume and training intensity. Volume is how much training you do, and intensity is how hard you work during the workout. You should be sure that the system you set up lets you manipulate these two variables independently. Also you have to decide how to measure these things and what units to use.

As an example of how to manipulate volume and intensity, consider an athlete training for an event that is 20 weeks away. She may decide to spend 8 weeks in a base-building phase to develop aerobic capacity. She designs this phase to feature a gradual increase in volume, from a low volume the first week, of perhaps 6 hours, to a very high volume of 25 hours by the end of 8 weeks, but all at a fairly low intensity. Next she may plan a second phase of perhaps 6 weeks focusing on raising her lactate threshold. This would feature more work at a moderate intensity, near her threshold, so she had better plan to reduce the volume accordingly, to perhaps 50 percent of her peak (25 hours) volume. In her planning, this athlete elects to gradually shift the volume and intensity levels from the first phase to the second.

Now, 14 weeks into her plan, she decides on a 4-week sharpening phase that emphasizes speed work—high-intensity training that she knows she could not maintain for the entire 20 weeks. Phasing in this increased intensity, she phases out still more of the volume, down to eight hours per week, to allow herself adequate recovery between hard workouts. For the final 2 weeks, she phases out the high-intensity training and keeps the volume low, "tapering" to a well-rested state in preparation for the event. This is just one example, of course, intended to show how coaches and athletes work with the concepts of volume and intensity and the relationship between them. The point is to be sure that your planning methods and tools deal with these concepts as well.

Training Volume

Training volume can be measured in distance, such as miles (usually miles per week), or in time (hours per week). Choose a measurement that you are comfortable with, but make sure it fits the training you will do. If you use cross-training or are training in multiple sports, such as in triathlon training, use time as the volume measure so you can get a value for the total training volume in all activities combined.

Training Intensity

Training intensity can be measured by speed or pace, by perceived effort, by heart rate, or by an abstraction of these called percent effort. It can be expressed, for planning purposes, as a percentage of your capability, such as "percent of 5K pace." Your choices depend on the training you will do. Again, for multiple activities, consider using percent effort, where an all-out effort is 100 percent. Your heart rate readings can easily be converted to this measure, and it is flexible enough to accommodate all types of workouts.

Dedicated athletes often find their specific heart rates for limits such as their anaerobic threshold, and may convert heart rate values to percent $\dot{V}O_2$max for more accuracy. This requires at least one session of testing in a sports medicine lab. But to those who want the best results, precise knowledge of a few beats per minute can be significant. This is especially true in workouts designed to take you to the limit of a certain energy system.

You can choose any measure for training volume and training intensity that works for you. There is no universally accepted method. Whatever measure you choose, you should be able to select a value in that scale for all your workouts, including the cross-training ones. If possible, use an indicator that you can get objective data about—in other words, one that you can measure with a monitor, stopwatch, or other instrument. Another approach is to record the workout data in a form that is directly derived from your indicators. For example, convert heart rate workout data into percent effort based on your known lactate threshold, and convert pace or speed data into percent effort based on your known best pace. Now both types of workouts have a common unit for intensity: percent effort. This way, when performing the workout you can get feedback from your heart monitor or speedometer or other tool and can tell whether you are doing the workout at the intensity and volume you had planned. Also, when you log that workout, you can record the specifics and later compare your "planned versus actual" in terms of both volume and intensity.

Most coaches deal with the variables of volume and intensity in some calendar unit, usually a week. The individual workouts in that week each get a percentage of the planned weekly volume. Likewise, each workout's intensity can be related to an overall intensity for the week, although this is less straightforward. Sophisticated systems such as the PC Coach Training Series software will do this for you mathematically, following the principles of the coach you select (fig. 10.3). Otherwise you will have to use your own ideas and perhaps use an approximation. If you are setting up your own training, you will want to incorporate at least a way to specify weekly training volume in your plan, as well as training intensity on at least an approximate level.

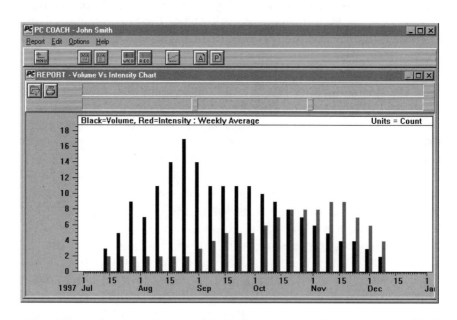

Figure 10.3 An example of periodized training volume.

Performance Evaluations

The goal in keeping records is to discover whether a given plan produces good results. To determine this, you need a solid, objective way to tell whether you are improving. This is called a performance evaluation. Evaluation workouts serve an important purpose, giving us a chance to see how our training and fitness are improving (or not) so we can either get a boost of encouragement or find out that we need to make adjustments. You will need to find or invent an evaluation workout and should plan to do it at periodic intervals so that later on you can see whether your plan has been working for you.

Surprisingly, race performance is often not the best evaluation. The results can be skewed by too many external factors: temperature, altitude, difficulty of the course, crowded race conditions, the level of competition, or the importance you give to the race. The best idea is to identify an evaluation workout, specifically designed for that purpose, that you can do privately under controlled conditions. Just be sure your instruments actually report the data you need to obtain.

You can be creative in devising performance evaluations using your heart monitor. One method, called the MAF test (Maximum Aerobic Function) is described in *Training for Endurance* by Dr. Philip Maffetone. In this test, you run or bike for a specified distance while keeping your heart rate precisely at a given number, which is down in your aerobic zone. Using the same heart rate each time you perform the test, you measure progress in your aerobic conditioning when your elapsed time drops in comparison to the elapsed time for earlier tests. Another test is to perform the same distance in the same time and measure your average heart rate. If you maintain the same pace at an increasingly lower average heart rate, you have a measure of progress in aerobic conditioning that you can quantify.

Evaluation of your speed in short sprints may also be important for your goals. This is easy to measure as a time value. Even with speed tests, you can use your monitor creatively, measuring the time it takes your heart to recover afterward, or the recovery rate you reach in a certain number of minutes after the sprint.

You may want several different tests in order to measure your progress in different areas. For example, you may want to measure improvements in sprinting speed as well as in cardiovascular fitness if both are a part of your ultimate goal. Don't expect to test both of them with the same evaluation. Create a separate test for each component.

When choosing your evaluation workout, also decide on the frequency. Whether you perform it every two, three, or four weeks, it is important to be consistent.

Neutralize differences in external factors like temperature, wind, and terrain by using the same track at the same time of day, such as morning when it's less windy. Make "all things equal" within yourself by consistently getting good rest the night before.

Personal Stats

This is the third category of data you can measure and record. Body weight, percent body fat, resting heart rate, and overall feeling (on a scale of 1 to 10, for example) are the most common and useful. Some people record their hours of sleep and sleep quality, but for most of us, that could be summed up as overall feeling. If diet is important to you, you can record daily caloric intake and perhaps more details such as percentages of fats, carbohydrates, and proteins. The important thing is to try to use items that can be objectively measured (the scale doesn't lie) or at least that can be recorded as a number, so you can graph out the results. Copious notes covering the details of your diet or sleep are fine if that is fun for you, but for most of us they are not necessary in order to get good information, and most people don't have the patience to look back at this information as a training tool.

You can gain a lot of information from recording your resting heart rate, and it is easy to obtain. Just stay in bed and count your heartbeats for 60 seconds before you get up in the morning. Do that two or three times per week, and you'll have another great feedback data item. You can see improvements in your fitness as your resting rate drops and be forewarned about impending problems when you notice a sudden spike. This indicates the onset of a cold or other illness or is a sign that you are becoming overstressed by your training. In either case, spotting it early and reducing your training effort for a day or two can help get you back quickly and avoid injuries and other similar disasters.

Pulling Together Your System

Now you have identified what data you can gather with the tools you have, and we have covered the basic ingredients of a measurable training system. Next I want to show you several options that you can use to set up your own system. These vary from the simple things anyone can do to sophisticated systems an aspiring athlete will want to use. The more data you gather, the more time you will spend dealing with the information, but the more accurate you can become in planning and analyzing. Any method you use, even the simplest, should share some fundamental ideas. I'll cover these again and then give you some possible systems.

First, find something that is objectively measurable with an instrument, even if it is just elapsed time. The combination of time and heart rate is best, with the addition of split and lap times for races and interval sessions. Use these measurable items as the basis for your planning effort so you can tell whether or not you are following the plan.

Second, plan your training and log your data with later analysis in mind. This means working in terms of volume and intensity and working in calendar units such as a week. It also means recording the volume and intensity of your workouts in such a way that you can look back at these values. Roll up the total weekly volume and graph it out. Graph out your intensity for each workout so you can see it. You can graph these as planned values, and as time moves along, can compare the planned values to your actual numbers. If possible, use a software tool such as PC Coach to do all this—it's much more time effective than putting it down on paper.

Third, have each of these three categories represented: training data, performance evaluation, and personal stats. Don't overlook the important information you can gather from low-tech items like the bathroom scale and the clock beside your bed.

Refer to table 10.1 for a description of three different approaches to a planning and monitoring system. These show reasonable data-gathering efforts in a simple system, a more detailed method, and a still more detailed method, which would normally coincide with an increasing degree of commitment in the athlete. The following example shows how these elements might fit into a day in the life of a nonprofessional athlete.

TABLE **10.1**	**Several Options** **for Data Monitoring**

Simplest method

Training data (planned and actual)

- Training volume—elapsed time or total distance, rolled into hours per week.
- Training intensity—in the measurement of your choice. If your tools allow, consider planning the volume and intensity as time spent in different heart rate zones.

Performance evaluation

- A simple evaluation workout, performed every three to four weeks.

Personal stats

- Body weight and "how I feel," recorded once per week.

More detailed method

Training data (planned and actual)

- To items listed for the simplest method, add a breakdown of your volume and intensity from weekly totals to each workout.
- Details of races (splits) and high-intensity workouts such as intervals.

Performance evaluation

- Add separate evaluations for speed and fitness components.

Personal stats

- Body weight and "how I feel," recorded daily if possible.
- Resting heart rate, recorded daily or two to three times per week.
- Periodically check percent body fat.

Still more detailed method

Training data (planned and actual)

- Invest in a monitor that records and downloads a heart rate profile for the workout.

(continued)

TABLE 10.1	*(continued)*

Performance evaluation

- Include the items listed for the first two methods.
- Add a test designed to detect changes in your lactate turn point, or anaerobic threshold, as your training progresses.

Personal stats

- Add a diet component, such as a simple estimate of caloric intake.
- Consider a periodic test to detect changes in the relation of heart rate to percent $\dot{V}O_2$max, or changes in anaerobic threshold heart rate.
- Consider a blood workup; consult a physician for more about this.

Our athlete wakens each day and remains in bed for 30 seconds, counting resting heart rate pulses, timed by the bedside clock. He then gets up, weighs himself, and writes down the resting heart rate, body weight, hours of sleep, and sleep quality on a notepad by the scale. This has consumed a total of two minutes, and already he has more objective data than many pro athletes ever obtain. Two days ago, he saw a resting heart rate that was seven beats higher than normal, so he replaced the scheduled high-intensity workout with an easy day. Yesterday was an easy workout. Today he sees that his resting heart rate is normal again, so he will resume his plan.

Time for the workout: The schedule calls for a lactate threshold run, holding the lactate threshold heart rate for 30 minutes. He performs this at the track, knowing that besides being a great workout, it is a chance to evaluate his progress if he uses the same course each time. He completes the workout and writes down the exact time and distance, 16 laps in 30:28 (he prefers to finish a full lap).

Back home, he enters his time and distance for the last several workouts into the computer, as well as the resting heart rate and body weight data for the past week. He doesn't get on the computer every day, so he refers to his written notes. He opens a graph that shows his total training hours (volume) for each week and sees that although he substituted an easier workout two days ago, he is still on target for total volume according to his original plan. He notices happily that next week is a recovery week and calls for less volume. That will clear up any concerns of overtraining that the elevated resting heart rate may have indicated. Now he opens a graph that shows his pace for recent lactate threshold workouts. He can see that at the same heart rate, his pace had continued to become faster each time except during this last workout. Since he knows that he should expect a slight drop in performance during a hard training week such as this and that the real gains will appear after the recovery week, he is not concerned.

Looking at his training for the past several weeks in this graphical form, he knows that with the exception of a well-advised adjustment eliminating one hard workout, he has stayed on his plan and his body is responding as expected. He has confidence that the plan will lead him to his goal and so can enjoy the lighter week to follow without guilt or concern. He knows that he has trained within his ability, avoided injury, and is getting the best results he could expect for this season.

This example reflects several important points. First, the athlete uses data from different categories: training data, personal stats, and evaluation data. Second, these data tell him something important that he uses in order to adjust his plan or to continue with confidence. The data are an important part of the training method; they are not collected simply out of curiosity. Third, the time required for this daily and weekly management probably amounted to a total of 30 minutes for the week.

Conclusion

Experts agree that a training system is essential in order to make progress in sports. Training systems are as unique as the individuals who create them, and your own will reflect your personal interests. If carefully designed at the start, your training system can work well for you for years to come. I hope this discussion can serve as a starting point for you in setting up your own system. Here again are the key factors to consider in designing a practical system.

Be sure you can use your system for planning, logging, and analysis. Take a moment to consider whether the data you want to record are compatible with the tools you have at hand. If you need better tools, get them early on. Consider using your computer as a basis for your training system.

Try to incorporate some element from each of three categories: workout data, performance evaluations, and personal stats. For workout data, consider the "planned versus actual" approach. Be sure that whatever values you use can express all the different types of workouts you do. Be consistent about your performance evaluations so you can accurately measure your progress. Above all, be realistic about the amount of time and effort you want to spend, and plan your record-keeping system accordingly.

ABOUT THE CONTRIBUTORS

Roy Benson is an exercise physiologist and coach. He holds a master's degree in physical education, with emphasis in exercise physiology, from the University of Florida. He also has national certification as a fitness instructor from the American College of Sports Medicine. Currently, he is contributing editor for *Atlanta Sports and Fitness Magazine*, *Running Journal*, and *Running Times*. Benson has written two books: *Precision Running with Your Electronic Coach* and *The Runner's Coach, A Workout Workbook*. His "Coach Benson's Heart Rate Running" computer program was recently published by PC Coach of Boulder, Colorado. His coaching experience includes 36 years as a professional track and distance running coach. Benson is the owner and president of Running, Ltd., a company that operates Coach Benson's NIKE Running Camps, held each summer for seven weeks in Colorado, California, North Carolina, and Vermont. He is a pioneer in the field of private coaching and has over 100 adult clients.

Jay Blahnik is the 1996 IDEA International Fitness Instructor of the Year, a NIKE-endorsed athlete, and the national fitness spokesperson for Polar heart rate monitors. He appears in, choreographs for, and consults on many award-winning exercise videos, and his work has appeared in numerous publications, including *Shape*, *Fitness*, *Self*, and *Fit* magazines. An author, celebrity fitness trainer, and industry trendsetter, Jay holds a degree from Cal Poly in San Luis Obispo and travels the world presenting health, fitness, and motivational workshops through his company, Body Dynamics.

Jim Dotter holds degrees in history and computer science from the University of Oklahoma. He has worked as a programmer and programming manager for 15 years, developing software in the areas of telecommunications and data communications. In 1992 he founded Biometrics, Inc., a company dedicated to the creation of software tools for athletes and coaches. Jim lives in Boulder, Colorado, where he serves as president of Biometrics.

Frank J. Fedel is an exercise specialist and researcher at the Henry Ford Heart and Vascular Institute in Detroit, Michigan. He conducted the first research study to examine the cardiovascular responses of competitive in-line skaters during skating. He has been a competitive in-line skater since 1991 and has been a coach and team manager for Team EXTREME Fitness and Health Promotion Team since 1992. Fedel is a columnist for *Fitness and Speed Skating Times* and *Columbus Sports* and is coauthor of *Fitness In-Line Skating* and *The 1998 Exercise and Nutrition Calendar*. He is a member of the American College of Sports Medicine.

Joe Friel has trained adult endurance athletes, including amateurs and professionals, since 1980. He holds a master's degree in exercise science and is an Expert-level certified coach with USA Cycling. He is currently serving on the USA Triathlon Coaching Certification Committee. A nationally recognized authority on endurance training, he is a regular contributor to such publications as *VeloNews*, *Inside Triathlon*, *Performance Conditioning for Cycling*, *Masters Sports*, and *Racing West*, and he has written a weekly training column for the *Fort Collins Coloradoan* newspaper since 1981. He is the author of *The Cyclist's Training Bible* and *The CompuTrainer Workout Manual*. Joe competes in cycling, triathlon, duathlon, and running.

Therese Iknoian is a master walking instructor and nationally published freelance health and fitness writer. Therese holds a master's degree in kinesiology with an emphasis in exercise physiology from California State University-Hayward. She is a member of Team Polar and has developed walking programming for several companies, including NIKE, Side 1, and Rockport. Therese is a contributing editor for *Walking* magazine, and her writing has also appeared in *Parenting*, *Self*, *Women's Day*, *Men's Health*, and *Women's Sports and Fitness*. She has written two books, *Fitness Walking* (1995) and a more advanced guide, *Walking Fast* (1998). She is an ACSM-certified Health/Fitness Instructor, a gold-certified ACE (American Council on Exercise) instructor, and a nationally ranked race walker. She is also certified as a coach and official by USA Track and Field.

Timothy J. Moore is president of Exercise Science, Inc., a health and fitness consulting company. He holds a master's degree in exercise physiology and a doctorate in health education. He is certified by the National Strength and Conditioning Association as a strength and conditioning specialist, as a personal trainer through the American Council on Exercise, and as an exercise test technologist from the American College of Sports Medicine. He is also a certified health education specialist. As a coach and trainer, he has worked with nationally ranked junior athletes, collegiate All-Americans, top professionals, and world champion senior competitors. As a triathlete, he participated in the Tri-Fed/USA National Amateur Triathlon Championships. His articles on health and fitness have appeared in such publications as *Women's Sports and Fitness*, *Triathlete*, *Inside Triathlon*, *The Physician and Sportsmedicine*, and *The National Strength and Conditioning Association Journal*. In addition, Dr. Moore has served as a fitness editor for *Shape* and as a member of the Advisory Board for the American Running and Fitness Association.

Wayne L. Westcott is fitness research director at the South Shore YMCA in Quincy, Massachusetts, and he is a strength training consultant for numerous national organizations, such as the American Council on Exercise, the National Sports Performance Association, and the National Youth Sports Safety Foundation. He is the editorial advisor for *Shape, Prevention, Club Industry, Men's Health, American Fitness Quarterly,* and *Nautilus* magazines, and he is the author of several fitness books, including *Building Strength and Stamina* (1996) and *Strength Training Past 50* (1998). Dr. Westcott received his PhD in physical education from The Ohio State University in 1977. He received the Lifetime Achievement Award from IDEA in 1993 and the Healthy American Fitness Leader Award from the President's Council on Physical Fitness and Sports in 1995.

ABOUT THE EDITOR

Edmund R. Burke, PhD, began working with HRMs in 1983, when he used these small electronic devices to prepare the U.S. cycling team for the Los Angeles Olympic Games. Over the years he's written numerous articles on HRMs and has served as a national spokesperson for the Polar Precision Fitness Institute.

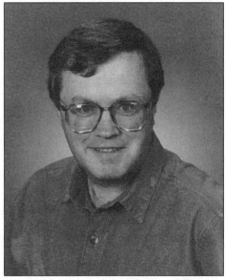

Dr. Burke has written or edited 11 books on health, fitness, and cycling, including *Serious Cycling* and *Complete Home Fitness Handbook.* The executive editor of *Cycling Science* and managing editor of *Performance Conditioning for Cycling,* he has also written extensively on cycling physiology, training, nutrition, health, and fitness for *Winning Magazine, MTB Magazine, NORBA News,* and *Bicycling.* He consults with several companies in the areas of cycling, fitness equipment design, nutritional products, and fitness programs.

Dr. Burke holds a doctorate in exercise physiology. He's a fellow of the American College of Sports Medicine, and he serves as vice president of research for the National Strength and Conditioning Association, with whom he's certified as a strength and conditioning specialist. Dr. Burke is also a professor in and director of the exercise science program at the University of Colorado at Colorado Springs, where he lives with his wife, Kathleen. In his leisure time Dr. Burke enjoys mountain biking, walking, and reading.

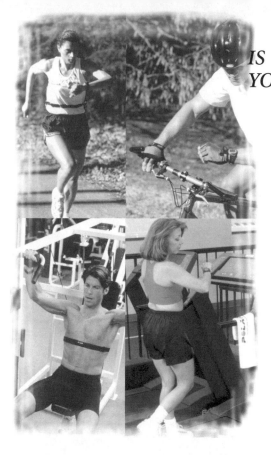

IS YOUR

Heart

In your

EXERCISE?

Determination alone is not enough to reach your performance goals. You need to exercise at the right intensity level.

Your heart rate is the most efficient indicator of exercise intensity.

Exercising

Too Easy — Initial benefit and then no further improvement.

Too Hard — Overtraining, risk of injury, exercise burnout.

Just Right — Efficient use of training time and the realization of your goal.

A Polar Heart Rate Monitor gives you a continuous display of your heart rate, making it easy to track your intensity during exercise. Put your heart in your training. It's the key to success!

A Polar Heart Rate Monitor is the most important piece of exercise equipment you will ever own!

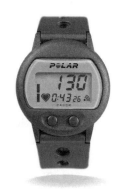

PolarPacer®

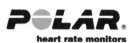

heart rate monitors